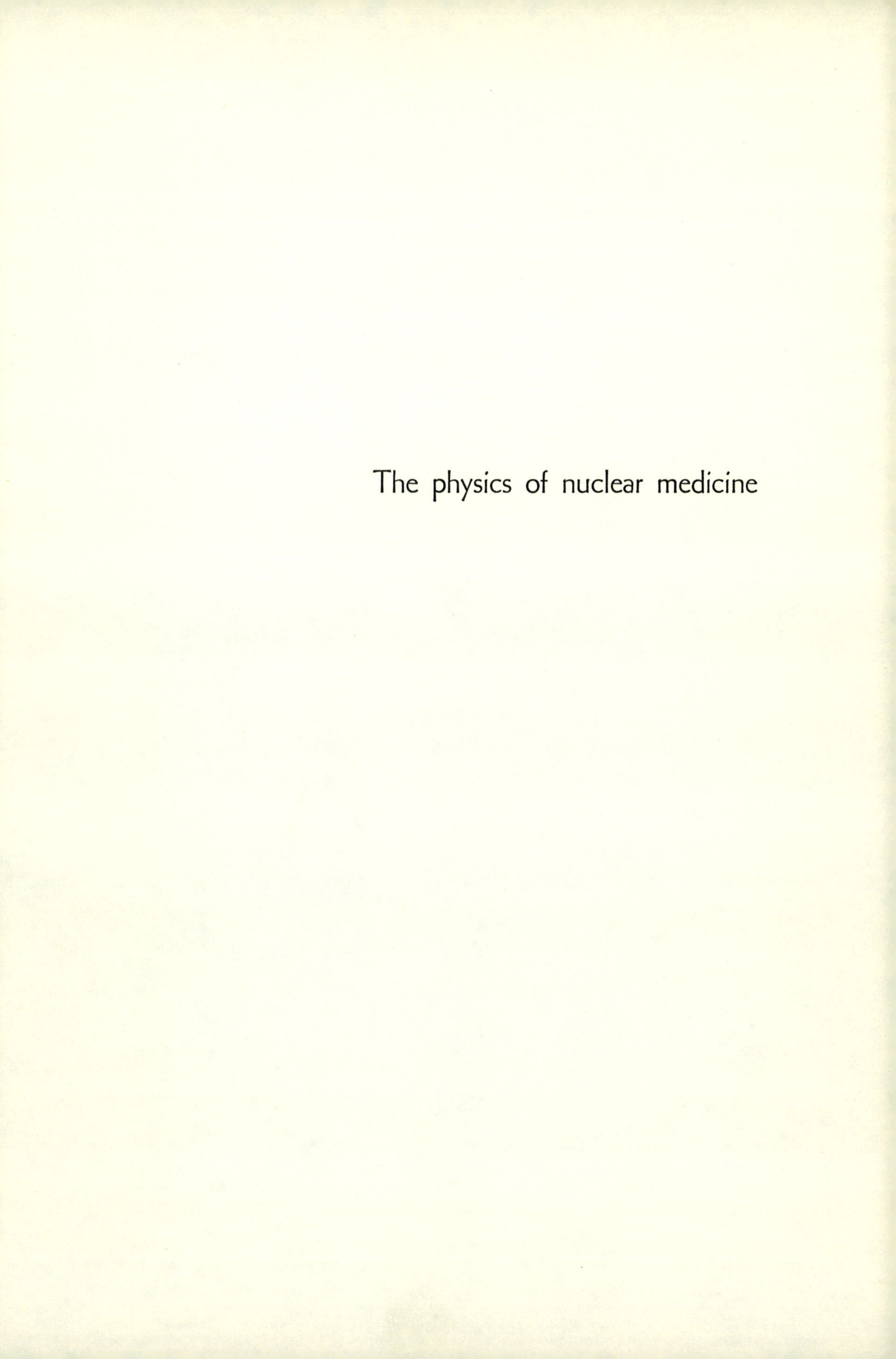

The physics of nuclear medicine

An introduction to
# The physics of nuclear medicine

By

## Paul N. Goodwin, Ph. D.

**Associate Professor of Radiology (Physics), and
Chief, Radiological Physics,
Albert Einstein College of Medicine,
Bronx, New York**

and

## Dandamudi V. Rao, Ph. D.

**Assistant Professor of Radiology (Physics),
and Director of Health Physics,
New Jersey Medical School
Newark, New Jersey**

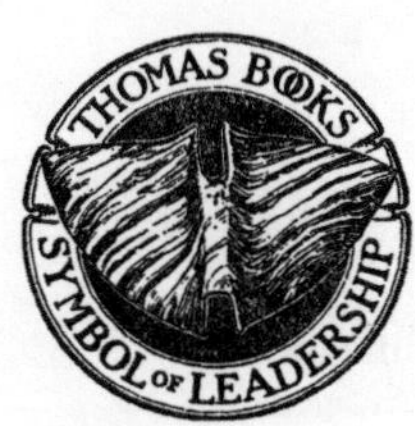


**CHARLES  C  THOMAS  •  PUBLISHER**
Springfield  •  Illinois  •  U.S.A.

*Published and Distributed Throughout the World by*
CHARLES C THOMAS • PUBLISHER
BANNERSTONE HOUSE
301-327 East Lawrence Avenue, Springfield, Illinois, U.S.A.



© *1977, by* CHARLES C THOMAS • PUBLISHER
ISBN 0-398-03569-5
Library of Congress Catalog Card Number: 76-8935

*With* THOMAS BOOKS *careful attention is given to all details of
manufacturing and design. It is the Publisher's desire to present
books that are satisfactory as to their physical qualities and artistic
possibilities and appropriate for their particular use.* THOMAS
BOOKS *will be true to those laws of quality that assure a good
name and good will.*

*Printed in the United States of America*
*N-1*

**Library of Congress Cataloging in Publication Data**

Goodwin, Paul N
    A introduction to the physics of nuclear medicine.

    Includes index.
    1. Nuclear medicine. 2. Medical physics. I. Rao, Dandamudi
V., joint author. II Title. III. Title: The physics of nuclear
medicine. [DNLM: 1. Nuclear medicine. 2. Nuclear physics. 3.
Physics. WN440 G657i 1976]
R895.G58          616.07'57          76-8935
ISBN 0-398-03569-5

# Preface

The physician who enters the field of nuclear medicine often finds that he has forgotten most of the physics to which he was exposed in college. Yet, in order to appreciate both the advantages and the limitations of nuclear imaging, he must understand the basic principles of radioactivity and radiation detection. This book presents those principles in as elementary a way as possible. Thus no attempt has been made to be comprehensive, but rather only that material is presented which will enable the physician to understand the equipment and the techniques used in his specialty. In addition, brief descriptions are given of some of the newer types of detectors and gamma cameras. We believe that these instruments, while not yet fully developed or widely available, will soon have a major impact on the field of nuclear medicine and that the physician who wishes to keep abreast of his specialty should understand the physical principles behind them.

The presentation is based on our experience in teaching physics to radiology residents, other M.D.'s, and nuclear medicine technologists. As an aid to self-study, problems and questions are included at the end of each chapter. These questions are of the multiple-choice type, so that the reader may determine if he has understood the subject matter.

Nuclear medicine technologists should find that this book covers most of the physics material for which they are held responsible on their certification exams. Also, this book may be of use to medical students who have the opportunity to take an elective in nuclear medicine, since an understanding of the basic principles and equipment will make their exposure to the field more interesting and profitable.

The authors would like to acknowledge advice and assistance from a number of persons who helped in preparing this book. In particular, we thank Professor K.S.R. Sastry, University of Massachusetts, for critical reading of the manuscript. Dr. Rao thanks Dr. M. Frendlich for his valuable criticism, Mrs. Vera Korda for her excellent typing, and his wife for her assistance. Dr. Goodwin thanks Dr. Leonard Freeman for helpful suggestions, Edith Ross, Joyce Rush, and particularly his wife, for secretarial assistance.

P.N.G.<br>
D.V.R.

# Foreword

There are many quotations which have become so cliched due to repetition that they lose all impact. A few, however, express so much truth that they still serve a purpose. One of these is the old adage that one must learn to walk before one can run. To do other than this is just about impossible. This is particularly applicable to the field of Nuclear Medicine, where persons who attempt to practice it as physicians or to perform procedures as technicians without understanding the physical principles involved could not expect to be able to define the limitations of their methods, select the appropriate studies, or to be able to properly use, care for, and calibrate their instrumentation. Without the knowledge of the basic physics, one would have to function by rote methodology, depending upon "cook book" procedures and interpreting studies through empiric recognition. Such a situation shortchanges the patient and places the physician treating that patient in jeopardy.

This book presents, in a simple and concise form, the physics necessary "to learn how to walk." No attempt has been made to inform the reader of the facts that do not relate directly to the studies or to the instruments which the practitioner will have to use. Some of the mathematics may seem detailed but working through the examples is not difficult, and the reader should at least know how his or her consulting or visiting physicist comes up with the magic numbers needed for new procedures or for health safety purposes. In addition, these types of calculations turn up with disturbing frequency on Board and Certification examinations.

Having spent considerable time teaching Nuclear Medicine principles to physicians, technicians, and students, I welcome this book. It clearly answers a need as a text for the physics lectures for students, residents, and technologists. In addition, it stands by itself as a self-study text for those in the field who need to walk leisurely and carefully through its pages in order to better compete in the Nuclear Medicine race.

MELVIN H. FREUNDLICH, M.D.
*Program Director of Nuclear Medicine;*
*Clinical Associate Professor of*
*Radiology and Medicine, College of*
*Medicine and Dentistry, New Jersey*
*Medical School, Newark, New Jersey*

# Contents

# The physics of nuclear medicine

# A review of elementary mathematics

**1**

To clearly explain physics without mathematical ideas is difficult. Although every attempt has been made to minimize the mathematical formalism, inescapably exponents and logarithms will be dealt with throughout this book. Therefore these mathematical ideas need to be discussed before going on to the physics of nuclear medicine.

## POWERS AND EXPONENTS

WHOLE NUMBERS. Supposing $y$ is any number and $m$ is its exponent which can be any positive whole number, then

$$y^m = y \times y \times y \ldots \ldots \ldots \ldots m \text{ times.} \tag{1.1}$$

Thus, $3^4 = 3 \times 3 \times 3 \times 3$ or $5^3 = 5 \times 5 \times 5$.

Also,

$$y^m \times y^n = y^{(m+n)}. \tag{1.2}$$

As an example, take

$$y = 3, m = 4, n = 2, \text{ then}$$
$$3^4 \times 3^2 = 3^6.$$

The division rule is

$$\frac{y^m}{y^n} = y^{(m-n)}. \tag{1.3}$$

Again, if $m = 4, n = 2,$ and $y = 3,$

$$\frac{3^4}{3^2} = 3^{(4-2)} = 3^2.$$

In equation $(1.3)$, if $n > m$, then the exponent is negative. For example, take $m = 2, n = 4, y = 3$, then

$$\frac{3 \times 3}{3 \times 3 \times 3 \times 3} = \frac{1}{3 \times 3} = \frac{1}{3^2}.$$

Use of equation $(1.3)$ gives

$$\frac{3^2}{3^4} = 3^{(2-4)} = 3^{-2},$$

suggesting

$$3^{-2} = \frac{1}{3^2}.$$

In general,

$$y^{-m} = \frac{1}{y^m}. \tag{1.4}$$

If $m = n$ in equation $(1.3)$, then

$$\frac{y^m}{y^m} = y^0 = y^{(m-m)}$$

But it is evident $y^m/y^m = 1$, therefore for any value of $y$,

$$y^0 = 1. \tag{1.5}$$

If $y^m$ is raised to power $n$, then

$$(y^m)^n = y^{(m \times n)}. \tag{1.6}$$

For $m = 4, n = 2$, and $y = 3$,

$$(3^4)^2 = 3^{(4 \times 2)} = 3^8.$$

FRACTIONS. The equations $(1.2)$, $(1.3)$, $(1.4)$, and $(1.6)$ are valid even though the exponents are fractions. Supposing $m$ is still a whole number, then $1/m$ is a fraction and

$$y^{\frac{1}{m}} = \sqrt[m]{y}. \tag{1.7}$$

If $m = 2$, then

$$y^{1/2} = \sqrt{y};$$

or $m = 4$,

$$y^{1/4} = \sqrt[4]{y}.$$

Also,

$$y^{\frac{m}{n}} = \sqrt[n]{y^m}. \tag{1.8}$$

For example, if $m = 2, n = 3$, then

$$y^{2/3} = \sqrt[3]{y^2}.$$

It also follows from above equations,

$$y^{1/2} = y^{0.5} = y^{5/10} = \sqrt[10]{y^5};$$

but

$$y^{1/2} = \sqrt{y},$$

which suggests that

$$\sqrt{y} = \sqrt[10]{y^5}.$$

LARGE AND SMALL NUMBERS. This book will deal with extremely large and small numbers. Therefore it is necessary to have an idea as to their magnitude. The velocity of light is a very large number, while the wavelength of yellow light is a very small number. How small or large are they? The velocity of light is known to be 30,000,000,000 cm/sec, i.e. 30 billion centimeters per second. The wavelength of yellow light is 0.000,058 cm, i.e. 58 times one millionth of a centimeter. Obviously these numbers are hard to deal with in this manner. A more convenient method using powers of ten is necessary.

To write the large numbers, positive whole-number powers of 10 are used.

$$10^m = \text{one followed by } m \text{ zeros.} \tag{1.9}$$

If $m = 0$, $10^0 = 1$ in agreement with equation (1.5),

$$10^1 = 10; \ 10^2 = 100; \ 10^6 = 1,000,000;$$
$$10^{12} = 1,000,000,000,000 \text{ and so on.}$$

Similarly, to write small numbers, negative whole-number powers of 10 are used.

$$10^{-m} = \text{A decimal point and } (m-1) \text{ zeros followed by } 1 \tag{1.10}$$

The value of $10^{-m}$ for $m = 0$ is still 1; $10^{-1} = 0.1$

$$10^{-2} = 0.01; \ 10^{-6} = 0.000,001,$$
$$10^{-12} = 0.000,000,000,001 \text{ and so on.}$$

Now the velocity of light and the wavelength of yellow light can be written in the above notation:

$$\text{velocity of light} = 30,000,000,000 \text{ cm/sec}$$
$$= 3 \times 10,000,000,000 \text{ cm/sec} = 3 \times 10^{10} \text{ cm/sec,}$$
$$\text{wavelength of yellow light} = 0.000,058 \text{ cm}$$
$$= 5.8 \times 10^{-5} \text{ cm.}$$

This notation also simplifies multiplication and division of numbers. For example, divide the velocity of light by the wavelength of the yellow light. If these numbers are not written in exponential form, it would be very difficult to carry out this operation.

$$\frac{\text{velocity of light}}{\text{wavelength of yellow light}} = \frac{3 \times 10^{10} \text{ cm/sec}}{5.8 \times 10^{-5} \text{ cm}}$$
$$= \frac{3 \times 10^{10} \times 10^5}{5.8} \text{ sec}^{-1}$$
$$= \frac{3}{5.8} \times 10^{15} \text{ sec}^{-1}$$
$$= 0.52 \times 10^{15} \text{ sec}^{-1}$$
$$= 5.2 \times 10^{14} \text{ sec}^{-1}.$$

Similarly the square of the velocity of light is

$$(3 \times 10^{10} \frac{cm}{sec})^2 = 3^2 \times (10^{10})^2 \ cm^2 \ sec^{-2}$$
$$= 9 \times 10^{20} \ cm^2 \ sec^{-2}.$$

## LOGARITHMS

Consider the equation

$$z = y^m.$$

Sometimes it is necessary to find the value of $m$, given $y$ and $z$. If $z = 100$ and $y = 10$, then

$$100 = 10^m.$$

In this case $m = 2$, which is not difficult to figure out. However, the exponent $m$ may not be a whole number, in which case it would be difficult to find the value of $m$.

For example, consider

$$12 = 10^m.$$

Since $10^1 = 10$ and $10^2 = 100$, the value of $m$ is somewhere between 1 and 2. In order to solve this kind of problem, the logarithm is very helpful. In general, the number $m$ in the equation:

$$m = \log_y z \tag{1.11}$$

is called the logarithm to the base $y$ of $z$. Here $y$ and $z$ can be any positive number, whole or fractional, except 0 and 1. In the example, $12 = 10^m$, the value of $m = \log_{10} 12$. Then the logarithm of 12 to the base 10 can be found.

The *common logarithms* tabulated in mathematical handbooks are usually to the base 10, which is found to be convenient to many calculations. The logarithm taken to the base $e$ is also useful sometimes. The value of $e$ is 2.71828. The logarithm taken to the base $e$ is called the *natural logarithm,* represented by ln. Which base should be used: 10 or $e$? For many calculations, base $e$ may be more convenient.

Consider the equation

$$z = e^m, \tag{1.12}$$

where $m$ is any positive or negative number. The value of $m$ that satisfies this equation can be obtained by taking logarithms on both sides:

$$\ln z = m \ln e.$$

But $\ln e = 1$, therefore

$$m = \ln z.$$

The natural logarithms and the values of the functions $e^{-m}$ and $e^m$ are tabulated in many mathematical handbooks. The availabilty of hand and desk calculators in many institutions makes these calculations even simpler.

The functions of the kind $e^{-m}$ and $e^m$ are important for understanding radioactive decay and absorption of radiation in matter. The value of the function $e^{-m}$ decreases from 1.0 when $m = 0$ very rapidly in the beginning and then slowly to zero as $m$ increases. The behavior of the function $e^m$ is just opposite to that of $e^{-m}$, i.e. increasing from 1 to infinity. The values of these functions are given in Table (1-I) for some chosen values of $m$.

*Example 1.1:* Calculate the value of $e^{-0.1} \times e^{0.1}$.

According to equation (1.2),

$$e^{-0.1} \times e^{0.1} = e^{(0.1-0.1)} = e^0 = 1.$$

This result is confirmed by using the values of exponentials.

From Table 1-I,

$$e^{-0.1} = .9048$$
$$e^{0.1} = 1.1052;$$

multiplication gives 1.

TABLE 1-I
VALUES OF $e^{-m}$ AND $e^m$

| $m$ | $e^{-m}$ | $e^m$ |
|---|---|---|
| 0 | 1 | 1 |
| 0.1 | 0.9048 | 1.1052 |
| 0.2 | 0.8187 | 1.2214 |
| 0.3 | 0.7408 | 1.3498 |
| 0.4 | 0.6703 | 1.4918 |
| 0.5 | 0.6065 | 1.6487 |
| 0.6 | 0.5488 | 1.8221 |
| 0.7 | 0.4966 | 2.0137 |
| 0.8 | 0.4493 | 2.2255 |
| 0.9 | 0.4066 | 2.4596 |
| 1.0 | 0.3679 | 2.7183 |
| 3.0 | 0.0479 | 20.0855 |
| 5.0 | 0.0067 | 148.4131 |
| 10.0 | 0.000045 | 22026.4658 |

## PROBLEMS AND QUESTIONS

1. $A^0 \times A^3$ is equal to
   (A)  0.
   (B)  $A^0$.
   (C)  $A^3$.
   (D)  1.

2. $4^{10}/4^8$ is equal to
   (A)  4.
   (B)  16.
   (C)  64.
   (D)  8.

3. $(A^4)^3$ is equal to
   (A)  $A^{64}$.

    (B)  $A^{12}$.
    (C)  $A^3$.
    (D)  $A^4$.

4. $1/(25)^{0.5}$ is equal to
    (A)  0.2.
    (B)  5.
    (C)  0.5.
    (D)  1.

5. $(25)^{1.5}$ is equal to
    (A)  5.
    (B)  25.
    (C)  37.5.
    (D)  125.

6. One light-year is 950,000,000,000,000,000 cm. In the exponential notation it is equal to
    (A)  $9.5 \times 10^{17}$.
    (B)  $9.5 \times 10^{18}$.
    (C)  $9.5 \times 10^{16}$.
    (D)  $95 \times 10^{17}$.

7. The electron charge is equal to 0.000,000,000,000,000,000,16 coulombs. It is equal to
    (A)  $1.6 \times 10^{-18}$.
    (B)  $1.6 \times 10^{-19}$.
    (C)  $1.6 \times 10^{-20}$.
    (D)  $1.6 \times 10^{-21}$.

8. Natural logarithms are taken to the base
    (A)  10.
    (B)  2.
    (C)  $e$.
    (D)  Any number not equal to zero or one.

9. The value of $e^{-m}$ varies from _______ to _______ with $m$.
    (A)  200, infinity
    (B)  one, zero
    (C)  one, infinity
    (D)  one, $e$

10. The value of $e^{m}$ varies from _______ to _______ with $m$.
    (A)  zero, infinity
    (B)  one, zero
    (C)  one, infinity
    (D)  one, $e$

# 2

# The structure of matter and the nature of radioactivity

In order to unravel the laws of nature, scientists follow a systematic approach called the *scientific* or the *inductive* method. This is essentially a three-step process: (1) Observe or experiment systematically and note the regularities. (2) Develop a theory or a model to explain the observed facts. (3) Predict from the model and test for its validity experimentally. If the theory explains all the known facts and if its predictions are found to be true experimentally, one could say that the particular model best represents the reality.

It may be necessary to modify the model to explain new experimental observations. Sometimes the modified model might fail to explain new discoveries, thus requiring a new model or a theory. If the theory is successful for many years, it becomes a *law* of nature. But one can never say that the law is absolute because any new experimental evidence might force the law to be modified or abandoned. Therefore one can only say that the theory is good enough to account for all the observed phenomena.

In the early nineteenth century, in order to explain the chemical behavior of many known elements, Dalton proposed the atomic hypothesis, which postulated:

1. All matter consists of discrete particles called atoms. They are the smallest units of matter and cannot be divided or changed.
2. The atoms of the same element are identical in all respects and different elements have atoms different in weight.
3. The combination of atoms of different elements results in chemical compounds.

This theory with some changes was able to explain all the observed phenomena, old and new, until the discovery of radioactivity by Becquerel in 1896 and the subsequent discovery of the electron by Thomson in 1897. A study of the properties of the electron revealed that it carries a charge and that it is very light, lighter than the smallest atom known. It became apparent that the atom must have an internal structure. Several atomic models were postulated to attempt to explain these new experimental observations. It was not until 1913, however, that Bohr suggested a model which finally explained these and later observations. This model, with some minor changes, is still in use today.

## THE ATOM

The hypothesis of Dalton, which stated that all matter consists of molecules made up of specific combinations of atoms, is still true. Atoms, in turn, are made up of some other smaller particles. Atoms consist of a central *nucleus* surrounded by *electrons* orbiting around the nucleus, as shown in Figure 2-1. It is a pattern similar to the planets moving around the sun. The electrons are negatively charged and carry very little mass while the nucleus contains most of the atomic mass and carries positive charge.

The mass of an electron is $9.1091 \times 10^{-28}$ gm. The charge of the electron is negative and has been found to be $1.6 \times 10^{-19}$ coulombs. This figure has become the unit of electrical charge, and all charges are multiples of the electron charge. Briefly, one can say that electrical charge occurs in discrete amounts.

The electrons in the atom move around the nucleus in definite orbits, or *shells*. The various orbits are characterized by a *quantum number*, n, which may take on the values of 1, 2, 3. . . . . as shown in Figure 2-1. The number of electrons possible in a given orbit is limited. There can be no more than $2n^2$ electrons with the same quantum number n. For an $n = 1$ orbit there can be only two electrons. Electrons which have the same quantum number are equivalent and belong to the same shell. The shells are denoted by the letters K, L, M, N . . . . for $n = 1, 2, 3, 4$ . . . . respectively. Thus, in the K shell which has a quantum number equal to 1, there can be a maximum of two electrons, while there are eight electrons in the L shell.

Nucleus. The nucleus is made up of particles called *protons* and *neutrons*. The charge of the proton is equal in size, but opposite in polarity to that of an electron. Since the atom is electrically neutral, the number of protons in a nucleus must be the same as the number of electrons surrounding the nucleus. The proton mass is $1.6725 \times 10^{-24}$ gm. The other member of the nucleus, the neutron particle, is electrically neutral and weighs $1.6748 \times 10^{-24}$ gm. The neutrons and the protons are much heavier than the electrons

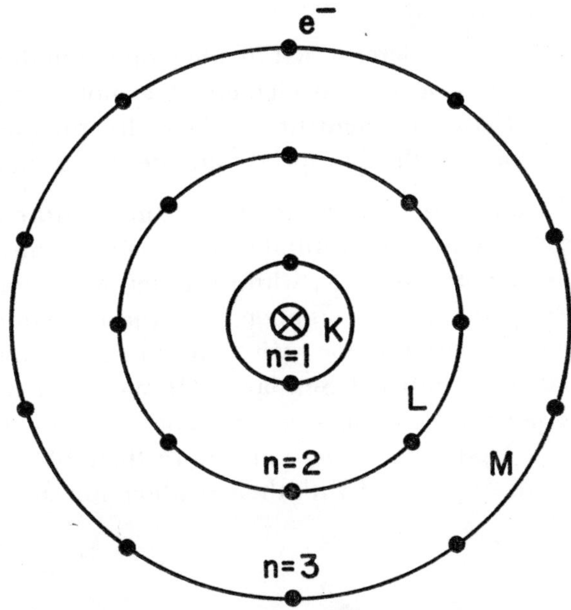


Figure 2-1. The structure of an atom.

and therefore the nucleus comprises almost all of the atomic mass. Either of the nuclear particles, i.e. neutrons and protons, are called *nucleons*.

The number of protons in the nucleus of the atom is the *atomic number* denoted by the letter Z. This number determines the element which the atom represents. For example, the simplest atom, hydrogen, has one proton in the nucleus and one electron orbiting in the nearest shell, the K shell. Therefore, the atomic number of hydrogen is 1. The helium atom has two protons in the nucleus and two electrons in the K shell. Its atomic number is 2. However, the lithium atom, with atomic number 3, has the third electron in the L shell since there cannot be more than two electrons in the K shell.

The neutrons are electrically neutral and are designated by the letter N. The number of neutrons present does not affect the atomic number, nor does it affect the number of electrons in the shells. It does change the atomic weight, however. The total number of neutrons and protons, i.e. the nucleons, in the nucleus is called the *mass number,* usually denoted by the letter A. In the case of hydrogen with only one proton in the nucleus, the mass number is 1, the same as the atomic number. But the helium nucleus with two protons and two neutrons in the nucleus has the mass number 4. Thus, each known atom is characterized by the atomic number Z, the mass number A and the neutron number N.

The specific element is determined by the atomic number. The addition of neutrons to a nucleus of a given element does not change the chemical behavior or the identity of the element. Symbolically, the nuclear species are identified as an element with appropriate atomic, neutron, and mass numbers as in $_Z X_N$ where X is the symbol for the element. More commonly, it is simply written as $^A X$. The proton number or atomic number is already determined by the element symbol X, while the neutron number can be obtained by subtracting the atomic number from the mass number, i.e. $N = A - Z$. For example, $^1H$ stands for hydrogen with mass number 1, atomic number 1 and neutron number 0. Similarly $^4He$ stands for helium with two protons and two neutrons in the nucleus. The structure of some simple atoms are shown in Figure 2-2. There are more than 100 elements known, and these are given in Appendix I with their symbols and atomic numbers.

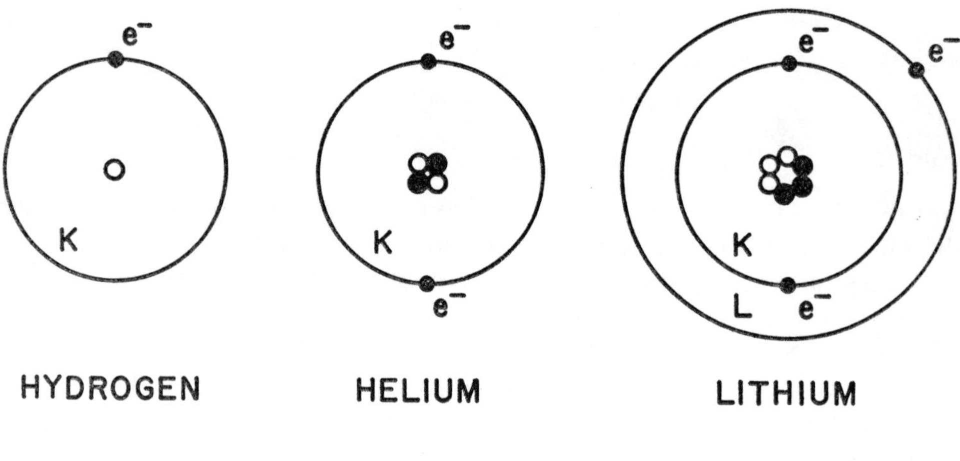


Figure 2-2. The structure of some simple atoms.

Certain elements are found to be composed of atoms having chemically identical properties but different weights. These are atoms whose nuclei have the same atomic number Z and therefore the same number of protons, but different number of neutrons N and hence different mass number A. Such atoms are called *isotopes*.

*Example 2.1:* Of the nuclides $^{131}$I, $^{130}$I, $^{130}$Xe, $^{132}$Cs, find the atoms with isotopic properties.

$^{131}$I:     $Z = 53$, $A = 131$, $N = 78$
$^{130}$I:     $Z = 53$, $A = 130$, $N = 77$
$^{130}$Xe: $Z = 54$, $A = 130$, $N = 76$
$^{132}$Cs: $Z = 55$, $A = 132$, $N = 77$

The atoms with the same Z, but different A and N values are $^{131}$I and $^{130}$I, which therefore are isotopes.

*Isobars* are those atoms with the same mass number A, but different Z and N. *Isotones* are atoms with the same neutron number N, but different Z and A numbers. If all the atomic, mass, and neutron numbers are the same, and if their radioactive properties are different, such species are called *isomers;* these will be discussed in Chapter 3. Isomers are usually denoted by m following the mass number in the superscript, e.g. $^{99m}$Tc.

*Example 2.2:* What are the isobars and isotones of the nuclides given in example 2.1?

Isobars:  Same A, therefore $^{130}$I, $^{130}$Xe
Isotones:  Same N, therefore $^{130}$I, $^{132}$Cs

ATOMIC AND NUCLEAR DIMENSIONS. The atom is very small. The radius is of the order of $10^{-8}$ cm. The space occupied by the nucleus in the atom is extremely small. The radius of the nucleus is of the order of $10^{-12}$ cm. Since much of the atomic weight is due to the small nucleus, the density of the nucleus is extremely high.

Since like charges repel and unlike charges attract, then one might wonder why the protons in the nucleus, all having positive charge, do not repel each other. For that matter, the negatively charged electrons in the orbits should also repel each other. If this principle held true, the protons in the nucleus would try to break apart. The basic postulate of the present atomic model is that an atom possesses a number of states and that the usual laws of electrodynamics are not valid for the particles in *stationary states.* That means there cannot be an attractive or repulsive force between the particles as long as they are in the stationary state. The nucleons are held together in the nucleus by a special strong short-range attractive force. When a proton lies beyond this short range, it will be repulsed by the nucleus.

If all the orbital electrons in the atom were to fall into the nucleus, the size of the atom would be $10^{-12}$ cm instead of $10^{-8}$ cm, a decrease in size by a factor of $10^4$. Then, the diameter of the earth would be less than a mile rather than approximately 8,000 miles.

## ENERGY AND MATTER

There are various forms of energy among which are mechanical, kinetic, and potential energy. Regardless of what the form of energy is, the total energy must be conserved. This is a basic law of physics. The unit of energy in the gm-cm-sec system is the *erg,* but it is not convenient to use this unit in atomic and nuclear physics. Instead, the term *electron volt,* usually denoted as eV, is used to express the atomic and nuclear energies. This is the energy acquired by an electron falling through a potential difference of one volt. The conversion factor from one unit to the other is

$$1 \text{ eV} = 1.6 \times 10^{-12} \text{ ergs.}$$

KeV and MeV stand for thousand electron volts and million electron volts, respectively.

Thus

$$1 \text{ keV} = 1.6 \times 10^{-9} \text{ ergs}$$
$$1 \text{ MeV} = 1.6 \times 10^{-6} \text{ ergs.}$$

ELECTROMAGNETIC RADIATION. A good example of electromagnetic radiation is visible light. The velocity of light, usually denoted by $c$, is constant and is equal to about $3 \times 10^{10}$ cm/sec or 186,000 miles/sec in a vacuum. It travels in a wavelike motion as shown in Figure 2-3.

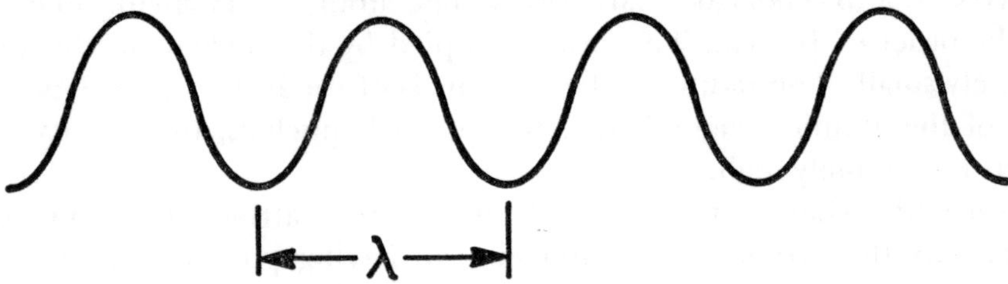

Figure 2-3. An illustration of wave motion.   The wavelength is the distance between two crests, or two valleys.

A wave is always associated with a wavelength denoted by $\lambda$, and a frequency $\nu$ with which it oscillates. The velocity of a wave is equal to the product of the wavelength and the frequency. Since the velocity of an electromagnetic wave is equal to the velocity of light, then

$$\lambda\nu = c = 3 \times 10^{10} \text{ cm/sec.} \tag{2.1}$$

The above equation can be used to calculate the frequency, knowing the wavelength or vice versa. Therefore either of these will specify the property of the wave, although $\lambda$ is used most often. The frequency increases as the wavelength decreases.

*Example 2.3:* The wavelength of green light is about $5 \times 10^{-5}$ cm. Calculate the frequency.

$$5 \times 10^{-5} \text{ cm} \times \nu = 3 \times 10^{10} \frac{\text{cm}}{\text{sec}}$$

$$\nu = \frac{3 \times 10^{10}}{5 \times 10^{-5}} \text{ sec}^{-1}$$

$$\nu = 6 \times 10^{14}/\text{sec}$$

The electromagnetic spectrum consists of waves whose wavelengths vary from many meters (radiowaves) to $10^{-13}$ cm or less (cosmic radiation). The electromagnetic radiations of interest to this book are those having wavelengths from $10^{-6}$ cm to $10^{-10}$ cm. It may be convenient to express such short wavelengths in terms of Angstrom units (Å).

$$1 \text{ Å} = 10^{-8} \text{ cm}$$

For example, the wavelength of green light is 5000 Å and that of X rays is of the order of an Angstrom unit.

Although electromagnetic radiations are considered as waves traveling with the velocity of light, they also behave as particles. Because they carry energy but no mass, electromagnetic radiations are also called *photons*. The amount of energy *(E)* carried by a photon depends on the frequency $\nu$, and therefore upon the wavelength $\lambda$. The energy of the photon can be obtained from the equation

$$E = h\nu, \tag{2.2}$$

where $h$ is Planck's constant:

$$h = 6.6 \times 10^{-27} \text{ erg-sec.}$$

The energy of a photon increases with its frequency. From equation (2.1), $\nu = c/\lambda$. Substituting for $\nu$ in equation (2.2), one obtains

$$E = \frac{hc}{\lambda}. \tag{2.3}$$

Thus, the energy is inversely proportional to the wavelength, which means the energy increases with decreasing wavelength. Although the photons have no mass, they have momentum equal to $h\nu/c$.

*Example 2.4:* Calculate the energy of green light.

The frequency is $6 \times 10^{14}/\text{sec}$. (See example 2.3)

$$E = (6.6 \times 10^{-27} \text{ erg-sec}) \times (6 \times 10^{14}/\text{sec})$$
$$= 39.6 \times 10^{-13} \text{ ergs.}$$

But $1 \text{ eV} = 1.6 \times 10^{-12}$ ergs, so

$$E = \frac{39.6 \times 10^{-13} \text{ ergs}}{1.6 \times 10^{-12} \text{ ergs/eV}}$$

$$E = 2.475 \text{ eV.}$$

If the wavelength of the photon is known, the equation (2.3) can be used to calculate the energy. It is a good exercise for the reader to try to obtain the following simplified equation for the energy of the photon whose wavelength is expressed in Angstrom units by substituting for $h$ and $c$ in equation (2.3) and by converting the energy to keV.

$$E(\text{keV}) = \frac{12.4}{\lambda(\text{Å})} \tag{2.4}$$

The wavelength of a photon can also be calculated if the energy is known from the above equation.

*Example 2.5:* Calculate the energy of the photon whose wavelength is $10^{-9}$ cm.

$$\lambda = 10^{-9} \text{ cm}$$

$$\lambda(\text{Å}) = \frac{10^{-9} \text{ cm}}{10^{-8} \text{ cm}} = 10^{-1} = 0.1$$

$$E(\text{keV}) = \frac{12.4}{0.1} = 124$$

The energy of the photon is 124 keV.

ATOMIC MASS UNIT. The mass of the atom and its constituent particles is so small that one must define a unit to express the mass of atomic particles. For this purpose the carbon atom with atomic number 6 and mass number 12 is taken as a standard. The atomic mass unit is then defined as the weight of a $^{12}$C atom per nucleon. According to Avogadro's hypothesis, 12 gms of $^{12}_{6}$C contain $6.0225 \times 10^{23}$ atoms. Then one atom of $^{12}_{6}$C weighs 12 gm/(6.0225 $\times 10^{23}$). The weight of one $^{12}_{6}$C atom per nucleon is.

$$\frac{1}{12} \times \frac{12 \text{ gm}}{6.0225 \times 10^{23}} = \frac{1}{6.0225 \times 10^{23}}$$
$$= 1.66044 \times 10^{-24} \text{ gm.}$$

Therefore, one atomic mass unit is equal to $1.66044 \times 10^{-24}$ gm. It is important to express mass units at least up to five decimal places.

*Example 2.6:* Express the mass of the electron, proton, and neutron in atomic mass units (amu).

$$\text{Electron: } \frac{9.1091 \times 10^{-28} \text{ gm}}{1.66044 \times 10^{-24} \text{ gm/amu}} = 0.0005486 \text{ amu}$$

$$\text{Proton: } \frac{1.6725 \times 10^{-24} \text{gm}}{1.66044 \times 10^{-24} \text{ gm/amu}} = 1.007263 \text{ amu}$$

$$\text{Neutron: } \frac{1.6748 \times 10^{-24} \text{ gm}}{1.66044 \times 10^{-24} \text{ gm/amu}} = 1.008648 \text{ amu}$$

EQUIVALENCE OF ENERGY AND MATTER. It was believed until 1905 that mass, like energy and momentum, would be conserved in all processes. Then it became difficult to explain certain experimental observations. For example, the mass of the nucleus was found to be less than the sum of the masses of the individual nucleons, which means that mass is not conserved in the formation of the nucleus. This loss of mass is explained by Einstein's postulate that matter is only a form of energy and that mass and energy can be converted into each other according to the formula

$$E = mc^2 \qquad (2.5)$$

where $m$ is the mass and $c$ is the velocity of light. Thus, the law of conservation of energy includes the conservation of mass. The observed mass discrepancy in the formation of the nucleus can be explained as the energy equivalent required to hold the nucleons together in the nucleus. It is called the *binding energy,* and is radiated away in the formation of the nucleus.

Now it is possible to express the atomic mass unit in terms of energy according to equation (2.5):

$$\text{amu} = (1.66044 \times 10^{-24} \text{ gm}) \, (3 \times 10^{10} \frac{\text{cm}}{\text{sec}})^2$$
$$= 1.66044 \times 9 \times 10^{-24} \times 10^{20} \text{ erg}$$
$$= 1.4944 \times 10^{-3} \text{ erg.}$$

Since

$$1 \text{ erg} = 6.25 \times 10^{11} \text{ eV,}$$
$$\text{amu} = 1.4944 \times 6.25 \times 10^8 \text{ eV}$$
$$= 934 \times 10^6 \text{ eV}$$
$$= 934 \text{ MeV.}$$

If one takes a more exact number for the velocity of light ($2.997925 \times 10^{10}$ cm/sec), a more accurate value for the energy equivalent mass unit will be obtained as 931.5 MeV. In other words, $1.66044 \times 10^{-24}$ gms of matter is equal to 931.5 MeV of energy.

> *Example 2.7:* Calculate the rest energy of an electron, proton, and neutron.
>
> Taking the rest masses of these particles from Example 2.6, one obtains for an
>
> Electron: $0.0005486 \times 931.5 = 0.511$ MeV
> Proton: $1.007263 \times 931.5 = 938.26$ MeV
> Neutron: $1.008648 \times 931.5 = 939.55$ MeV.

> *Example 2.8:* A free neutron disintegrates eventually into a proton, an electron and a particle called a *neutrino.* The mass of the neutrino is almost zero and it is electrically neutral. It travels with the velocity of light. Use the law of conservation of energy to calculate the kinetic energy available for these product particles.
>
> Rest energy of neutron $= 939.55$ MeV
> Sum of the rest energies of the product

$$\text{particles} = 938.26 + 0.511 + 0$$
$$= 938.771 \text{ MeV}$$
$$\text{Difference in rest energy of the initial and}$$
$$\text{final particles} = 939.55 - 938.77$$
$$= 0.78 \text{ MeV}$$

## RADIOACTIVITY

RADIOACTIVITY OF NUCLEAR ORIGIN. The nuclei have discrete energy states or levels which are characteristic of the nucleus. The nucleus always attempts to be in a stable or ground state. It is possible to produce many unstable elements by bombarding stable elements with small particles such as neutrons, protons, electrons, etc. or by breaking heavy elements such as uranium into pieces of smaller unstable elements. The latter process is called *fission* and can only be performed in a nuclear reactor. These processes will be further discussed in Chapter 9.

All unstable isotopes attempt to reach a stable state through a process of decay which involves the emission of radiation. The spontaneous emission of radiation by the unstable nucleus is called *radioactivity*.

There are basically three kinds of radiations emitted by radioisotopes or radionuclides: $\alpha$ rays, $\beta$ rays, and $\gamma$ rays. Not all three radiations are emitted simultaneously by all radioactive nuclides. Some emit $\alpha$ rays, others emit $\beta$ rays, while the $\gamma$ rays are sometimes emitted with either $\alpha$ or $\beta$ rays. These and other decay processes will be considered in the next chapter.

The type and energy of the radiation emitted by a radionuclide is the specific property of that particular isotope and has nothing to do with the chemical behavior of the element. Another characteristic of radioactivity is that the radiations are emitted *isotropically*, i.e. with no preferred direction of emission.

RADIATIONS OF ATOMIC ORIGIN. The basic postulate of the atomic model is that an atom possesses a number of discrete stationary states. Every state is associated with an energy. When the system is in the lowest possible energy state, it is said to be in the *ground state*.

Consider, for example, the lithium $(_3\text{Li}^6)$ atom containing three electrons in the orbits. Two electrons will be in the K shell and one in the L shell. These are the lowest possible energy states for the electrons and therefore the $_3\text{Li}^6$ atom is stable and is in the ground state. Suppose one of the K electrons is knocked out by external means; then there will be only one electron in the K shell and one in the L Shell. The lithium atom is then said to be in the *excited state*. A system which is in an excited state eventually goes to the ground state. In our example, the L electron then jumps to fill the vacancy in the K shell. The energy difference between these two shells is emitted as radiation. The radiation emitted by atoms due to the transfer of electrons from higher shells to more stable lower shells is characteristic of the atoms and is therefore called *characteristic radiation.* The wavelength of the radiation emitted belongs to the x-ray region of the electromagnetic spectrum.

The electrons in the shells are bound. Energy equal to the binding energy must be supplied to remove an electron from a shell. The binding energy is highest for K electrons and decreases with the increasing shell number. The actual binding energy of the electrons in the shells depends on the atomic number Z. Because of this binding energy, the energy of the x ray photon emitted during the transition of an electron from the L shell to the K shell is actually equal to the difference of the K shell binding energy and L shell binding energy.

In atoms of higher atomic numbers, a greater number of shells are filled with electrons. In case of a K vacancy, a transition of electrons from any higher shell is possible to the K shell. The resulting x rays are called K x rays. If an L electron is ejected or jumps to the K shell, then the L vacancy will be filled by the transition of electrons from higher shells, emitting L x rays. This process, as illustrated in Figure 2-4, continues until the atom reaches its stable state of energy.

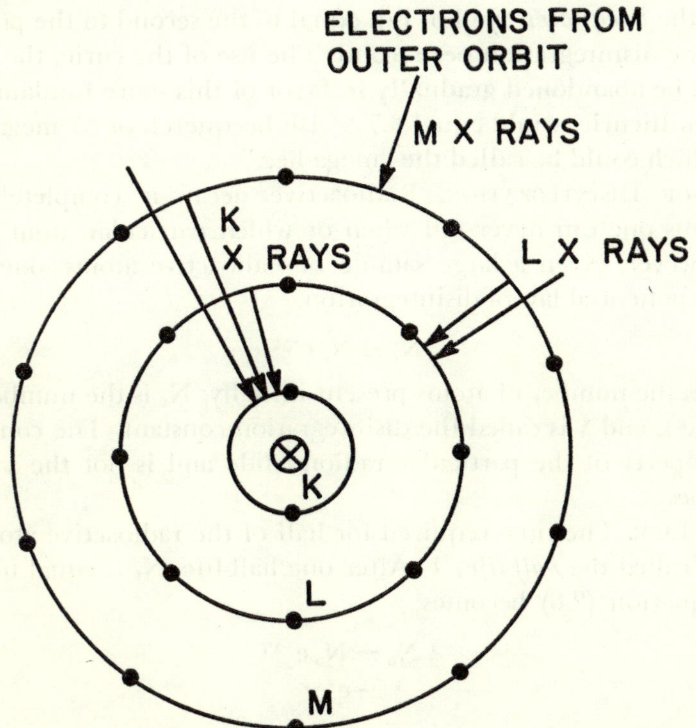


Figure 2-4. A diagram of an atom showing the shells.  Characteristic x rays are emitted due to the transition of electrons from higher orbits to lower orbits.

Sometimes it is possible that the energy of the characteristic x ray is given to an orbital electron whose binding energy is less than the energy of the x-ray photon. The electron is then ejected out with the kinetic energy equal to the difference of the x-ray energy and the electron-binding energy of the shell to which it originally belonged. Such electrons are called *Auger electrons.*

UNITS OF RADIOACTIVITY. The rate at which radionuclides disintegrate or the intensity of the radioactivity is called *activity.* The unit of activity is the curie, written as Ci, and originally defined as the amount of activity of one gram of radium in equilibrium with its decay products, approximately $3.7 \times 10^{10}$ disintegrations per second.

Activities of the order of curies are not used in nuclear medicine procedures. Therefore, smaller units, which are given below, may be used.

$$1 \text{ curie (Ci)} = 3.7 \times 10^{10} \text{ dis/sec}$$
$$1 \text{ millicurie (mCi)} = 3.7 \times 10^{7} \text{ dis/sec}$$
$$1 \text{ microcurie } (\mu\text{Ci)} = 3.7 \times 10^{4} \text{ dis/sec}$$
$$1 \text{ nanocurie (nCi)} = 3.7 \times 10 \text{ dis/sec}$$

The International Commission on Radiation Units and Measurements (ICRU) has recently recommended that the name of the unit for activity should be the *becquerel,* symbol Bq, equal to the second to the power minus one, i.e., one disintegration per second. The use of the curie, the millicurie, etc. should be abandoned gradually in favor of this more fundamental unit. Thus the millicurie would equal $3.7 \times 10^{7}$ becquerel, or 37 megabecquerel, (MBq), which could be called the "mega-bec."

LAW OF DISINTEGRATION. Radioactive decay is completely random, which means one can never tell when or which particular atom is going to decay. However, given a large sample of radioactive atoms, one finds they obey the exponential law of disintegration.

$$N_t = N_o\, e^{-\lambda t} \tag{2.6}$$

where $N_o$ is the number of atoms present initially, $N_t$ is the number of atoms after a time t, and $\lambda$ is called the disintegration constant. The constant $\lambda$ is a specific property of the particular radionuclide and is not the same for all radioisotopes.

HALF LIFE. The time required for half of the radioactive atoms present to decay is called the *half-life,* T. After one half-life, $N_t$ is equal to $\frac{1}{2} N_o$, and then the equation (2.6) becomes

$$\frac{1}{2} N_o = N_o\, e^{-\lambda T}$$
$$\frac{1}{2} = e^{-\lambda T}$$

Taking natural logarithm on both sides, the equation becomes

$$\ln \left(\tfrac{1}{2}\right) = -\lambda T$$
$$\ln 2 = \lambda T$$
$$0.693 = \lambda T$$
$$\lambda = \frac{0.693}{T}. \tag{2.7}$$

Thus, the disintegration constant can be calculated knowing the half-life of the radionuclide. The $\lambda$, from equation (2.7), can be substituted in equation (2.6) to obtain

$$N_t = N_o \, e^{-0.693t/T}. \tag{2.8}$$

Figure 2-5 illustrates the relationship between the activity and half-life. The fraction of activity remaining after n half-lives is $\left(\tfrac{1}{2}\right)^n$.

*Example 2.9:* The half-life of technetium-99m is 6 hours. Calculate the disintegration constant. From Eq. (2.7),

$$\lambda = \frac{0.693}{T}$$
$$T = 6 \text{ hours}$$
$$\lambda = \frac{0.693}{6 \text{ hrs}} = 0.1155/\text{hrs}.$$

*Example 2.10:* A shipment of 80 mCi of $^{99m}$Tc is received at 9 AM. One half of its activity is used immediately. Calculate the remaining activity at 3 PM the same day and at 9 AM the next day.

Remaining activity at 9 AM the same day $= (80 - 40)$ mCi
$$= 40 \text{ mCi}.$$

By 3 PM, the time elapsed $= 6$ hrs.
Since the half-life of $^{99m}$Tc is 6 hrs, the remaining activity at 3PM $= 40$ mCi $\times \tfrac{1}{2} = 20$ mCi.
By 9 AM, next day, the time elapsed $= 24$ hrs
$$= 4 \text{ half-lives of } ^{99m}\text{Tc}.$$

After 4 half-lives, the fraction of remaining activity is
$$\left(\tfrac{1}{2}\right)^4 = 1/16 = 0.0625.$$
The remaining activity $= 40$ mCi $\times 0.0625$
$$= 2.5 \text{ mCi}.$$

*Example 2.11:* What is the time required to reduce the initial activity of $^{99m}$Tc to less than 1 percent?
From the above example it is known that in 4 half-lives

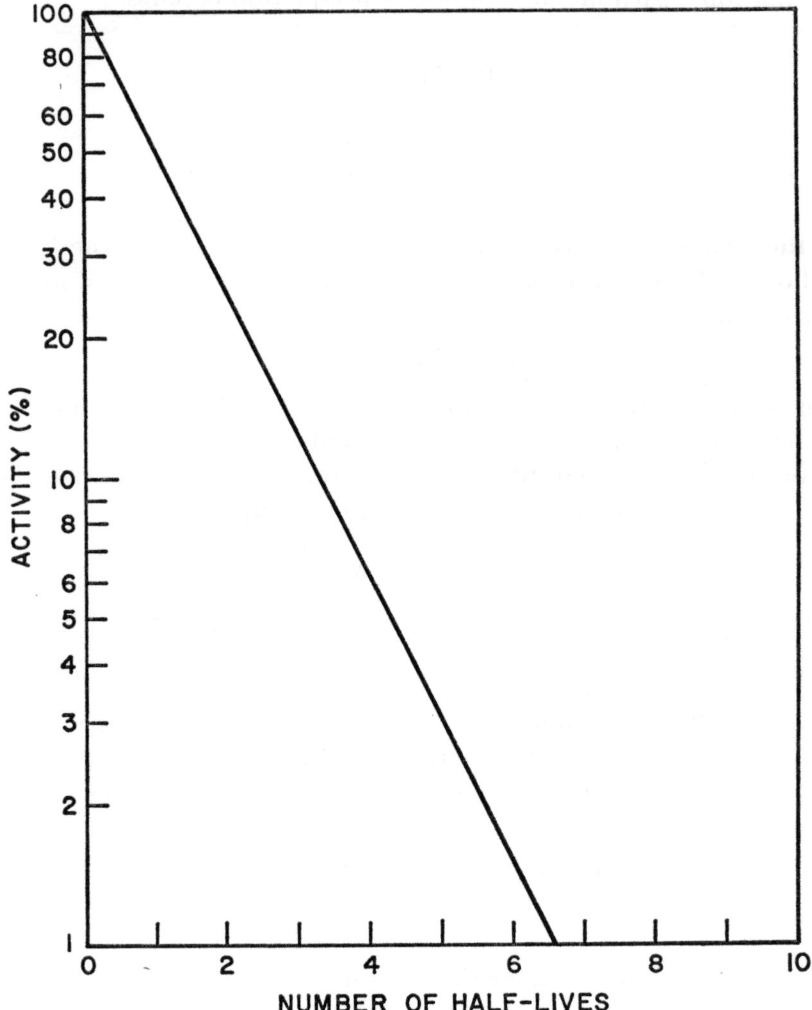


Figure 2-5. An illustration of the relationship between the activity and the half-life.

the remaining fractional activity is 0.0625 or 6.25 percent.

$$5T - 3.125\%$$
$$6T - 1.562\%$$
$$7T - 0.781\%$$

The activity after 7 half-lives is 0.78 percent.

Total time required is about $(7 \times 6)$ hours, or forty-two hours.

When a radioactive sample does not contain any stable isotopes of that element, it is said to be *carrier free*. Such radioisotopes are desirable for clinical use. *Specific activity* is the activity per unit weight of the radioactive sample. For carrier-free samples of radioactivity, the specific activity is very high. When used in regard to radioactive shipments, the term specific activity, or concentration, refers to the activity per unit volume of the isotope solution. The specific activity decreases with time due to the decay of the radioisotope.

> *Example 2.12:* Calculate the specific activity at the times given in example 2.10 if the total activity is contained in 10 ml of solution.
>
> 9 AM same day:  80 mCi in 10 ml
>
> $$\text{The specific activity} = \frac{80 \text{ mCi}}{10 \text{ ml}} = 8 \text{ mCi/ml.}$$
>
> 3 PM same day:  20 mCi in 5 ml
>
> $$\text{The specific activity} = \frac{20 \text{ mCi}}{5 \text{ ml}} = 4 \text{ mCi/ml.}$$
>
> 9 AM next day:  2.5 mCi in 5 ml
>
> $$\text{The specific activity} = \frac{2.5 \text{ mCi}}{5 \text{ ml}} = 0.5 \text{ mCi/ml.}$$

## PROBLEMS AND QUESTIONS

1. The atomic shell with quantum number n = 4 is the
   (A)  K shell.
   (B)  L shell.
   (C)  M shell.
   (D)  N shell.

2. The maximum number of electrons in the M shell is
   (A)  2.
   (B)  8.
   (C)  18.
   (D)  32.

3. The number of neutrons in $^{99}$Mo whose atomic number is 42, are
   (A)  99.
   (B)  57.
   (C)  42.
   (D)  141.

4. In the elements $^{99}$Tc, $^{99}$Mo, $^{100}$Tc, $^{97}$Nb, the isotopes are
   (A)  $^{99}$Tc, $^{99}$Mo.
   (B)  $^{99}$Tc, $^{100}$Tc.
   (C)  $^{99}$Tc, $^{97}$Nb.
   (D)  $^{99}$Mo, $^{97}$Nb.

5. The isobars in the above elements are
    (A) $^{99}$Tc, $^{99}$Mo.
    (B) $^{99}$Tc, $^{100}$Tc.
    (C) $^{99}$Tc, $^{97}$Nb.
    (D) $^{99}$Mo, $^{97}$Nb.

6. The isotones in the above elements are
    (A) $^{99}$Tc, $^{99}$Mo.
    (B) $^{99}$Tc, $^{100}$Tc.
    (C) $^{99}$Tc, $^{97}$Nb.
    (D) $^{99}$Mo, $^{97}$Nb.

7. The wavelength of 1.24 MeV photon is
    (A) 0.1 Å.
    (B) 0.01 Å.
    (C) 1 Å.
    (D) 0.001 Å.

8. The transition of an electron from M to K shell results in the emission of
    (A) M x rays.
    (B) L x rays.
    (C) K x rays.
    (D) K and L x rays.

9. The disintegration constant for $^{99}$Mo is 0.25 per day. The half-life is about
    (A) 0.25 day.
    (B) 6 hours.
    (C) 2.8 hours.
    (D) 2.8 days.

10. The time required to reduce the $^{99}$Mo activity to less than 1 percent is about
    (A) 3 days.
    (B) 6 days.
    (C) 10 days.
    (D) 20 days.

# 3

# Nuclear decay processes

In the previous chapter it was stated that all radioactivity represents an attempt by a nucleus to give up energy and thus reach a lower and more stable energy level. There are many ways in which a nucleus may lose energy. Since mass is a form of energy, a loss of mass, such as the ejection of a particle from the nucleus, results in a loss of energy. In addition, any particle which has both mass and velocity also has kinetic energy; thus the nucleus may lose energy by ejecting high-speed particles. One form of radioactive decay by a loss of mass is the ejection of two protons and two neutrons, bound together to form an alpha particle. Decay by alpha emission occurs only among the heavier elements. Since alpha particles travel only a few microns in tissue, and produce high internal radiation doses, they are of little interest in clinical nuclear medicine, and will not be further discussed here. Other methods by which a nucleus can lose energy will now be described.

## NEGATIVE BETA DECAY

In this decay process, a neutron ($n^0$) within the nucleus changes into a proton ($p^+$) plus an electron ($e^-$); the electron is immediately ejected from the nucleus as a high-speed "beta particle." This process may be diagrammed as shown in Figure 3-1. The horizontal lines indicate differences in energy levels; the diagonal line goes to the right because the process is an *increase* in the atomic number Z. Each beta process results in a definite loss of energy, known as the *transition energy*, but individual beta particles may have any energy from zero up to the transition energy. In each case, the difference between the beta particle energy and the transition energy is carried away by another particle, known as a neutrino $\nu$, which has no charge, virtually no mass, and is almost impossible to detect.

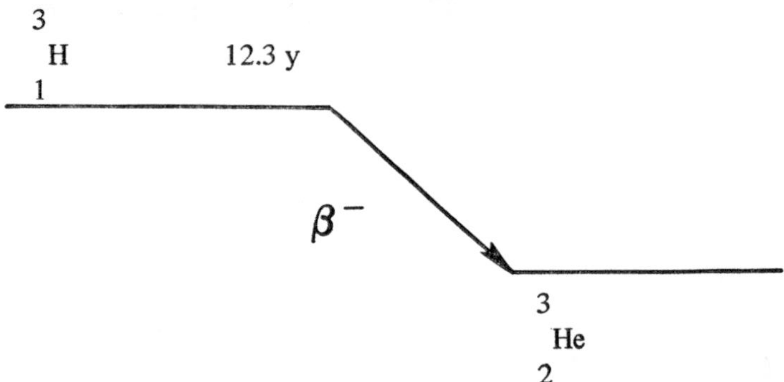

Figure 3-1. Decay scheme for a nuclide, $^3$H, which decays by simple $\beta^-$ decay.

For example, in the case of $^3$H, the transition energy is 18.6 keV, but the average beta particle energy is only 5.7 keV, or about 30 percent of the maximum. For most beta emitters, the average beta energy is between 30 percent and 40 percent of the maximum, or transition energy. The rest of the energy is carried away by neutrinos.

Thus in beta decay the nucleus loses both the energy equivalent of the electron mass and the kinetic energy associated with the high-speed electron and the neutrino. The neutron to proton ratio is also reduced.

Negative beta decay may be summarized by the relation:

$$n^o \rightarrow p^+ + e^- + \nu.$$

Beta particles have a range in tissue of only a few millimeters, so radionuclides which decay by pure beta emission are difficult to detect externally, and thus are not used for imaging procedures. However, some pure beta emitters, such as $^{14}$C and $^{32}$P are widely used as tracers in cases where detection can be performed by *in vitro* techniques.

## GAMMA EMISSION

Most radionuclides which decay by beta emission also emit gamma rays. The initial beta emission leaves the daughter nucleus in an excited state, so further energy is released in the form of one or more gamma rays. The diagram for this is shown in Figure 3-2 for a simple beta-gamma emitter, $^{203}$Hg. Here a beta particle is emitted, having a maximum energy of 213 keV, followed immediately by a gamma ray with an energy of 279 keV.

A more complex example is molybdenum-99, whose decay scheme is shown in Figure 3-3. Here any one nuclide may decay by beta emission to one of several possible energy levels, followed by a single gamma ray or a cascade of gamma rays to reach lower energy levels including that of technetium-99m, whose decay will be discussed later.

Other examples of beta-gamma decay are iodine-131, cesium-137, and gold-198. When beta-gamma emitters are administered internally, most of

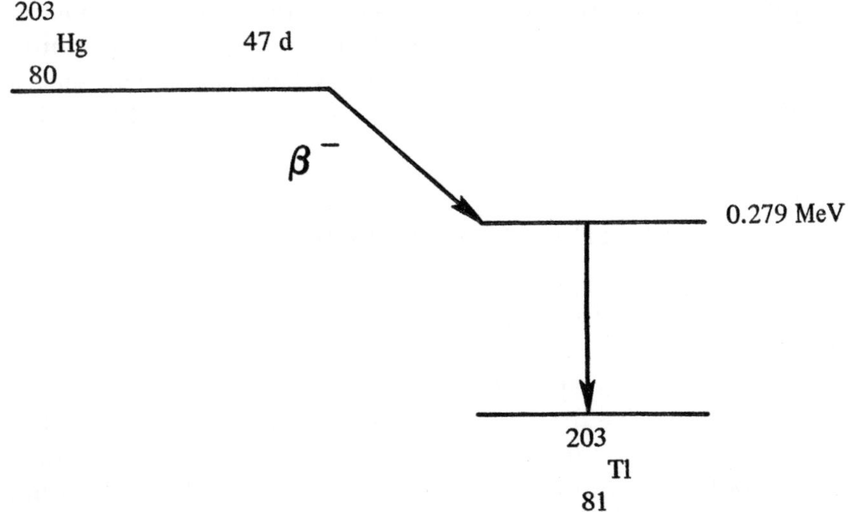

Figure 3-2. Decay scheme for a nuclide, $^{203}$Hg, which decays by simple beta-gamma decay.

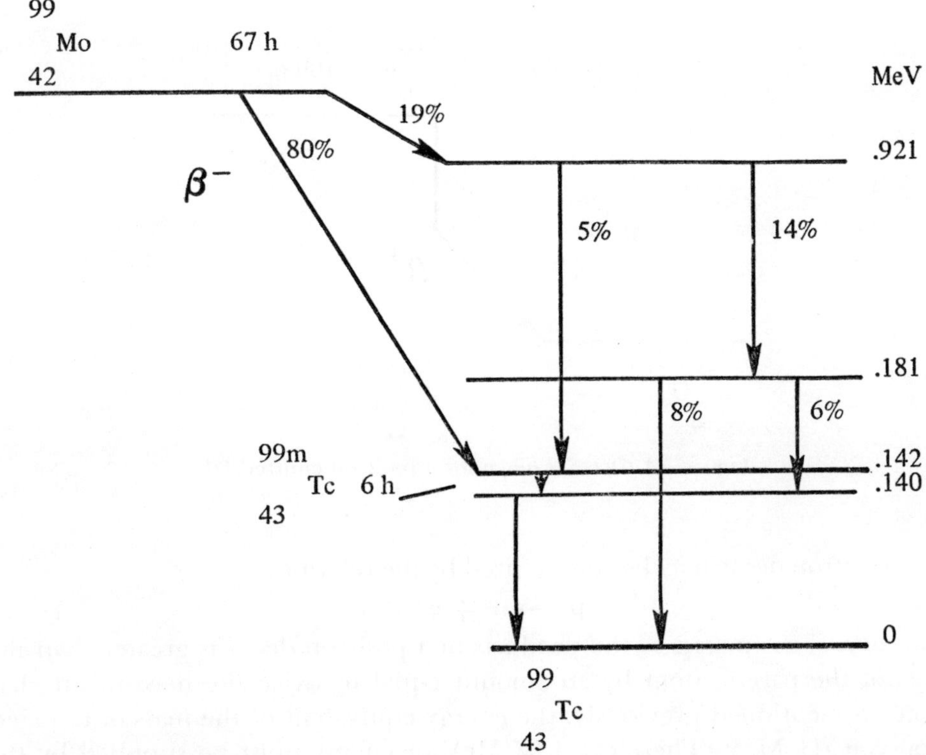

Figure 3-3. Simplified decay scheme for $^{99}$Mo. About 80 percent of the $^{99}$Mo nuclei decay by beta emission directly to $^{99m}$Tc. The remaining 20 percent decay is by beta emission to other energy levels, of which only the principle one is shown.

the radiation dose is contributed by the beta particles. Thus, to obtain maximum external detection for a given radiation dose, beta-gamma emitters are to be avoided if possible. In spite of this, many beta-gamma emitters, such as iodine-131, have been widely used because of their availability and ease of external detection.

## POSITIVE BETA (POSITRON) DECAY

If a nucleus has a higher proton-to-neutron ratio than is desirable for stability, then it is possible for a proton to change into a neutron plus a positive electron, called a *positron* $(e^+)$. This positron, which has the same mass as the electron but opposite charge, is immediately ejected as a high-speed beta particle. The diagram for positive beta decay is shown in Figure 3-4 for $^{18}$F. A diagonal line to the left is used to indicate a loss of atomic number, as well as a definite energy loss by the nucleus. Like electrons, positrons may be emitted with any energy from zero up to some maximum value. For each nuclear decay, the difference between this value and the energy of the positron is carried away by the neutrino.

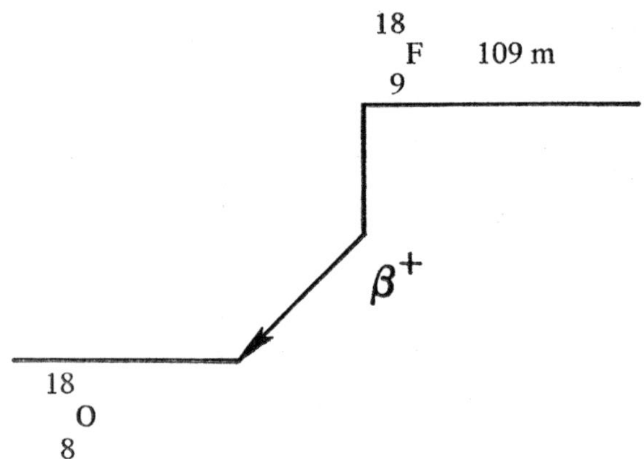


Figure 3-4. Decay scheme for a positron emitter, $^{18}$F.

Positron decay may be summarized by the relation:

$$p^+ \rightarrow n^o + e^+ + \nu$$

The sum of the masses of the products of a positron decay is greater than the mass of the parent atom by an amount equal to twice the mass of an electron. As mentioned previously, the energy equivalent of the mass of the electron is 0.511 MeV. Therefore 1.02 MeV of energy must be supplied by the parent nucleus before positron decay can take place. This 1.02 MeV energy drop is represented by the vertical line in Figure 3-4.

Positrons, like electrons, have ranges in tissue of only a few millimeters. The emitted positron immediately undergoes a number of collisions or deflections and loses its kinetic energy. As soon as it comes to rest, it unites with a negative electron. The rest masses of the two particles, which have a total energy equivalent of 1.02 MeV, are converted into two gamma rays of 0.511 MeV each, which are emitted in exactly opposite directions. Thus all positron emitters can be readily detected by a scintillation scanner or gamma camera; or use may be made of a positron detector consisting of two scanners or cameras on opposite sides of the source, connected so as to respond only when two gamma rays are simultaneously absorbed in opposite detectors.

As with beta-gamma emitters, most of the internal dose from positron emitters results from the beta particles, while the annihilation gamma rays make possible external detection. Because of the relatively high energy of the annihilation gamma rays, positron emitters may require considerable lead shielding. Other isotopes which decay by positron emission include carbon-11, nitrogen-13, and oxygen-15.

## ELECTRON CAPTURE

Another method by which a nucleus can decay is for the nucleus to capture one of its orbital electrons, usually one from the innermost, or K shell; thus this process is also known as "K capture." The captured electron combines with a proton in the nucleus to form a neutron, thus reducing the proton-neutron ratio. This may be written:

$$p^+ + e^- \rightarrow n^o + \nu$$

An example of a decay scheme for electron capture is shown in Figure 3-5, for $^{125}I$, which decays by electron capture followed by emission of a single gamma ray.

When an electron is removed from the K shell of an atom, the vacancy in the K shell is filled immediately by another electron, most probably from the L shell, but possibly from the M, N, or other outer shells. Since the K shell represents the most tightly bound state, an electron falling into a vacancy in the K shell will release energy equal to the difference between the K-shell energy and the L or other level from which it originated. This energy may be released in the form of a single photon, known as a *characteristic x ray,* since the energy levels are different for each element, and thus the photons are characteristic of that particular element. For medium and heavy elements, characteristic x rays have energies from about 20 to 100 keV, and thus may be a factor in shielding as well as in external detection of the radionuclide.

The energy which is available when a K-shell or L-shell vacancy is filled may also be transferred directly to an outer electron, causing it to be ejected

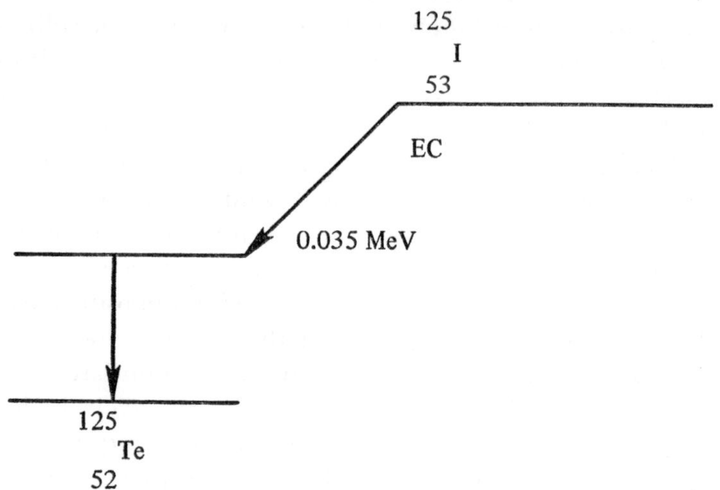


Figure 3-5. Decay scheme for a nuclide, [125]I, which decays by electron capture, followed by gamma emission. The K x ray emitted following electron capture is normally not shown on the decay scheme.

from the atom. These characteristic electrons, the Auger electrons, have definite kinetic energies (as discussed on page 20) and may be viewed as an alternative to characteristic x-ray emission. The fractional number of K characteristic x rays emitted per K vacancy is called the K *fluorescent yield,* and increases with increasing atomic number.

Thus radionuclides which decay by electron capture will emit x rays characteristic of the daughter nuclide, in addition to any gamma rays which may be emitted. These characteristic x rays may be used for external detection or gamma imaging. For example, in the case of [125]I, most of the emitted photons are characteristic x rays of 27 to 31 keV, while for [197]Hg, which decays by electron capture (EC) followed by gamma emission, most of the photons are characteristic x rays of 67 to 81 keV. Other radionuclides which provide useful K x rays following EC include erbium-165, with K x rays of about 50 keV, and thallium-201, with K x rays of about 70 keV.

## ISOMERIC TRANSITIONS

The process whereby a nucleus loses energy without a change in the proton-neutron ratio is known as an isomeric transition. The simplest form is the emission of energy in the form of a gamma ray. Most radionuclides which decay by beta-gamma emission emit beta particles followed immediately by a gamma ray. However, for some radionuclides the daughter nucleus may pause in the excited state before dropping to the ground state. If the pause is for a measurable length of time, then the nucleus is in a metastable state. An example of such a metastable radionuclide is $^{99m}$Tc, as shown in Figure 3-3. A metastable radionuclide may undergo an *isomeric transition,* that is, lose energy and drop to the ground state, in one of two ways: either by the emission of a gamma ray, as previously mentioned, or by transferring its energy directly to one of its orbital electrons, usually a K-shell electron. This process is known, rather inappropriately, as internal conversion. The electron then has too much energy and is ejected from the atom. The ratio of internal conversions to gamma rays is known as the conversion ratio; for $^{99m}$Tc it is about 0.1. When a K shell or L shell electron is ejected, another electron fills in the vacancy, resulting in the emission of characteristic x rays and Auger electrons. Thus radionuclides which decay by isomeric transition emit gamma rays, x rays, Auger electrons, and internal conversion electrons.

Some radionuclides, in addition to $^{99m}$Tc, which decay by isomeric transition are indium-113m and strontium-87m.

## QUESTIONS

1. The radionuclide $^{131}_{53}$I undergoes $\beta^-$ decay with a half-life of 8.1 days. The respective atomic and mass numbers of the daughter nucleus are
   (A) 53, 131.
   (B) 52, 130.
   (C) 54, 131.
   (D) 53, 130.

2. The atomic number of the product nucleus from $\beta^+$ decay
   (A) increases by 1.
   (B) decreases by 1.
   (C) does not change.
   (D) decreases by 2.

3. Beta particles emitted by a radionuclide
   (A) are monoenergetic depending on the nucleus.
   (B) will have many discrete energies depending on the nucleus.
   (C) will have a continuous energy spectrum that is the same for all beta emitters.
   (D) will have a continuous spectrum with a maximum energy characteristic of the radionuclide.

4. The neutrino is a particle
   (A) with almost no mass and carries charge equal to an electron.
   (B) with a mass equal to an electron and carries no charge.
   (C) with no rest mass and no charge.
   (D) like a neutron.

5. Internal conversion is the process in which
   (A) a proton is converted into a neutron inside the nucleus.

    (B) a neutron is converted into a neutrino and an electron.

    (C) a neutron is converted into a proton.

    (D) the excitation energy of the nucleus is used to eject an orbital electron.

6. Internal conversion process competes with

    (A) $\beta^-$ decay.

    (B) $\beta^+$ decay.

    (C) $\gamma$ decay.

    (D) none of the above.

7. The K fluorescent yield is

    (A) the number of characteristic K x rays emitted per K shell vacancy.

    (B) the fraction of photons emitted during isomeric transition.

    (C) the fraction of orbital electrons ejected during internal conversion.

    (D) the number of photons emitted in $\gamma$ decay.

8. For positron decay, the minimum energy difference between parent and daughter atoms must be

    (A) 0.51 MeV.

    (B) 1.02 MeV.

    (C) between 0 and 0.51 MeV.

    (D) between 0.51 and 1.02 MeV.

9. Positron decay competes with

    (A) $\alpha$ decay.

    (B) $\gamma$ decay.

    (C) electron capture.

    (D) internal conversion.

10. Isometric transition is that in which the parent and daughter nuclei

    (A) emit the same radiations.

    (B) have the same atomic and mass numbers.

    (C) are radioactive.

    (D) undergo $\beta^-$ decay.

11. A radionuclide X undergoes electron capture to the ground state of the stable nucleus Y. The expected radiations are

    (A) none.

    (B) positrons.

    (C) characteristic X rays and Auger electrons.

    (D) only Auger electrons.

12. The average energy of the electrons in $\beta$ decay is approximately

    (A) the same as the maximum energy.

    (B) one half of the maximum energy.

    (C) one third of the maximum energy.

    (D) one fourth of the maximum energy .

# 4

# The interaction of radiation with matter

Most radiations interact with matter by imparting energy to the matter in which they traverse. Radiations can be detected only if they interact with matter. For example, the neutrino particle described in the previous chapter is very hard to detect because its interaction probability in matter is extremely small. For this reason, these particles cannot cause significant damage to living material. Different kinds of radiation interact differently with matter and these differences are exploited in developing instruments to detect each kind.

The radiations of interest in nuclear medicine can be divided into two classes:

1. those having mass and charge such as electrons and positrons, and
2. electromagnetic radiation (no mass and no charge).

The neutron carries mass, but no charge and belongs to yet a different class. It can also interact in matter but it will not be discussed in this book.

The radiations emitted during a nuclear disintegration are alpha particles, electrons, positrons, and photons. The radionuclides decaying by the emission of alpha particles are not useful in nuclear medicine. However, they might have some value in radiation therapy. The interaction of radiations emitted during nuclear decay with matter is the subject of this chapter.

## ALPHA PARTICLES

Alpha particles are nothing more than helium nuclei which consist of two protons and two neutrons. The masses of the proton and the neutron in the nuclei are approximately the same and each particle is about 1800 times heavier than the electron. The rest mass of an electron is 0.511 MeV (remember that mass can be expressed in terms of energy according to Einstein's formula: $E = mc^2$). Since there are four nucleons in the alpha particle, the particle is 7200 times heavier than an electron and therefore the rest energy of the alpha particle is about 3600 MeV. Alpha particles are commonly emitted in the radioactive decay of the heaviest elements $(Z > 82)$. The kinetic energy of alpha particles emitted from the natural radionuclides varies from 4 MeV to 10 MeV, which is very small compared to the rest energy of the alpha particle. The velocities of the alpha particles at these kinetic energies range from 1 to $2 \times 10^9$ cm/sec. Although this velocity appears to be very high, these alpha particles can be absorbed by a sheet of paper.

The energy of alpha particles is lost by causing *ionization* in matter along their paths. Ionization is the process in which the incoming particle gives up energy by removing an electron from a neutral atom, thus producing an *ion pair*. The alpha particle continues to travel in matter until all the kinetic energy is used in this manner and eventually comes to rest. It then finds two free electrons to form a helium atom.

The range $(R)$ of the alpha particle in air at 15° C and 760 mm of mercury (atmospheric pressure) increases with increasing energy and can be calculated using the empirical formula

$$R = 0.318 \, E^{1.5} \text{ cm,} \tag{4.1}$$

in which $E$ is the energy of the alpha particle expressed in MeV. According to this formula, the 7.68 MeV alpha particle from $^{214}$Po will have a range in air of 6.77 cm. The range of alpha particles emitted by radionuclides is much less in solid matter. They cannot even penetrate the dead layer of the skin; therefore, there is little danger of external exposure to alpha particles from radionuclides. However, the radionuclides can be very dangerous if they are ingested or inhaled.

## BETA PARTICLES

Unlike alpha particles, beta particles are very light and have a continuous energy spectrum. The maximum energy available to the electron from nuclear decay is also called the *end point energy* which is a characteristic of the decaying radionuclide. The number of beta particles emitted with this maximum energy are very few. The accompanying neutrino carries no or very little kinetic energy when the electron energy is maximum. The electrons of atomic origin ejected by the internal conversion process are monoenergetic and should not be confused with the electrons of nuclear origin.

ABSORPTION OF BETA PARTICLES. Like alpha particles, electrons lose most of their energy ionizing atoms along their paths. However, the penetrating power of beta particles is high when compared to alpha particles. This is due to the higher velocity of the electrons which permits them to spend comparatively less time in the vicinity of an atom, thus reducing the probability of interaction. In addition, the electron has a single charge while the alpha particle bears two positive charges. For both of these above reasons the relative ionization caused by beta particles is low. For example, a 3 MeV beta particle produces four ion pairs/mm of path in standard air and travels about 1000 cm.

The absorption of beta particles emitted by radionuclides in solid matter is approximately exponential, occurring rapidly in the beginning and then slowly as the thickness of the matter increases. In other words, the number of beta particles decreases exponentially with increasing absorber thickness up to a point where all the particles are absorbed.

The maximum distance travelled by the beta particles, that is the range, depends on their energy and the density of the matter being traversed. The empirical formula used to obtain the range in unit density material is:

$$R = 0.546\, E_o - 0.16 \text{ cm} \tag{4.2}$$

where $E_o$ is the maximum energy of the beta particles in MeV emitted by a radionuclide. This formula gives the approximate range of beta particles in unit density matter such as water. For $E_o$ less than 500 keV, the above equation gives considerably different ranges and therefore it should be used only for higher beta particle energies. The range in any material whose density is not unity can be obtained by dividing the result obtained using equation (4.2) by the density of the absorber.

*Example 4.1:* The radionuclide phosphorus-32 emits beta particles whose maximum energy is 1.71 MeV. Calculate the maximum range of these particles in water, aluminum, and lead if the respective densities are 1, 2.7, and 11.34.

$$\text{Range in water} = 0.546 \times 1.71 - 0.16 = 0.774 \text{ cm}$$

$$\text{Range in aluminum} = \frac{0.774}{2.7} = 0.29 \text{ cm}$$

$$\text{Range in lead} = \frac{0.774}{11.34} = 0.07 \text{ cm}$$

Taking human soft tissue as unit density matter, the above example shows that phosphorus-32 beta particles can penetrate up to about 0.8 cm in depth.

BREMSSTRAHLUNG. For low-energy beta particles the energy loss in matter is completely by ionization. When high-energy beta particles are involved, a small fraction of the total energy is lost by another process of interaction. This other process occurs when an electron passes near an atomic nucleus of the absorber. The particle's direction of travel changes due to the attractive force between the negatively charged electron and the positively charged nucleus. This sudden change in the path causes the electron to lose energy by radiation which is known as *bremsstrahlung*. The fraction of energy lost by the electron in this process increases as the electron energy and the atomic number of the absorber increase. An approximate formula for the fraction of bremsstrahlung loss is given by

$$f_{br} = \frac{ZE_0}{3000}, \tag{4.3}$$

where Z is the atomic number of the absorber and $E_0$ is the maximum beta particle energy in MeV.

    *Example 4.2:* Calculate the energy loss by radiation for beta particles emitted by $^{32}P$ in aluminum $(Z = 13)$ and lead $(Z = 82)$. The maximum energy for the beta particles is 1.71 MeV. In aluminum,

$$f_{br} = \frac{1.71 \times 13}{3000} = 0.0075.$$

About 0.7 percent of the total energy, or 12 keV, is lost as bremsstrahlung radiation.
In lead,

$$f_{br} = \frac{1.71 \times 82}{3000} = 0.047.$$

The radiation loss is about 4.7 percent of the total energy, or 80 keV, which is about six times more than the loss in aluminum.

    Positrons. Since a positron is the *antiparticle* of an electron, the points discussed so far may be applied to positrons also. However, after all its energy is lost, the electron finds an electron-deficient atom and attaches itself to that atom, while the positron, being positively charged cannot do so. The positron combines with an electron which is almost at rest, the particles annihilating each other and giving out energy in the form of electromagnetic radiation. According to the principle of conservation of energy, the total energy produced is equal to the sum of the rest energies of the particles. The rest energy is equal to the rest mass of the particle. The rest mass of an electron or a positron is 0.511 MeV. Therefore the total annihilation energy is 1.022 MeV. Because both particles are almost at rest before annihilation, the total momentum is zero. The law of conservation of momentum suggests that the total momentum must also be zero after annihilation. Although photons carry no mass, they have momentum equal to $h\nu/c$. Then the annihilation energy cannot be emitted as a single photon of 1.022 MeV energy because in that case momentum is not conserved. Two photons of equal energy emitted in opposite directions would conserve momentum as well as energy. The two-photon annihilation process of a positron and an electron is summarized in Figure 4-1. One and three-photon annihilation processes are also possible

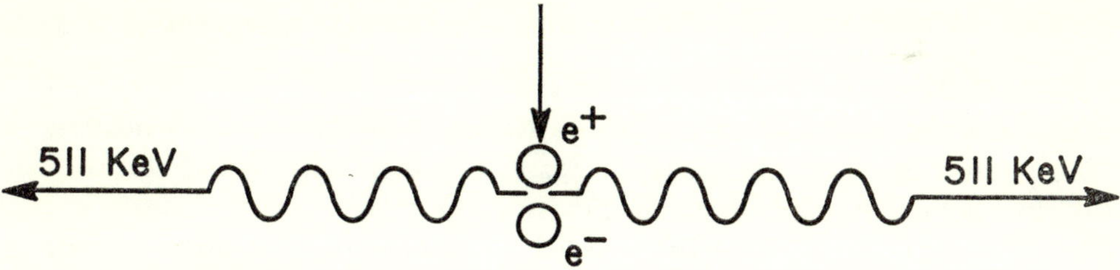


Figure 4-1. Annihilation of a positron with an electron leaves two photons of energy 511 keV going in opposite directions.

under certain favorable conditions, but they can be ignored for the purposes of this book.

The 511 keV photons resulting from annihilation will in turn interact with matter in an entirely different manner which will be discussed in the next section. The two photons of equal energy emitted in opposite directions are used for *coincidence* imaging, a technique which has some advantages over conventional imaging and will be discussed in Chapter 8.

## PHOTONS

Photons of nuclear origin are called gamma rays. When a nucleus is in an excited state, sooner or later the nucleus will go to a less excited state through the emission of gamma ray. In nuclear medicine one is primarily interested in the detection of gamma rays emitted by a suitable radionuclide given to a patient. Characteristic x rays from heavy Z elements are of atomic origin and can also be used for imaging. They are emitted either because of internal conversion or electron capture decay. The radionuclides iodine-125, erbium-165, mercury-197 and thallium-201 are good examples of nuclides which produce this kind of radiation.

It is very important to understand the interaction of photons in general with matter. Unlike beta particles, the gamma photons from the decay of radionuclides have discrete energies. All photons, no matter what their energy and origin, carry no mass or charge and travel with the velocity of light. The absorption mechanism of photons by matter is therefore different than that of charged particles.

Absorption by Matter. The absorption or attenuation of photons by matter is the result of photons interacting with the atomic electrons or nuclei. Consider a beam of monoenergetic photons whose intensity is $I$. A thin slab of matter whose thickness is $X$ is placed across the beam. If $\mu$ is the probability of interaction per unit distance, then the change in intensity is

$$-\Delta I = \mu I \Delta X \qquad (4.4)$$

The minus sign is to indicate the decrease in beam intensity. The constant $\mu$ is called the *attenuation coefficient*. The integration of equation (4.4) gives

$$I = I_o\, e^{-\mu x} \tag{4.5}$$

where $I$ is the intensity of the photons after going through a thickness X. The photon intensity therefore decreases exponentially as the thickness of the absorber increases, as shown in Figure (4-2).

The thickness of absorber needed to reduce the intensity to half its original value is called the *half-value layer* (HVL) or *half-thickness*. If 100 photons are incident, 50 of them will penetrate through the HVL without

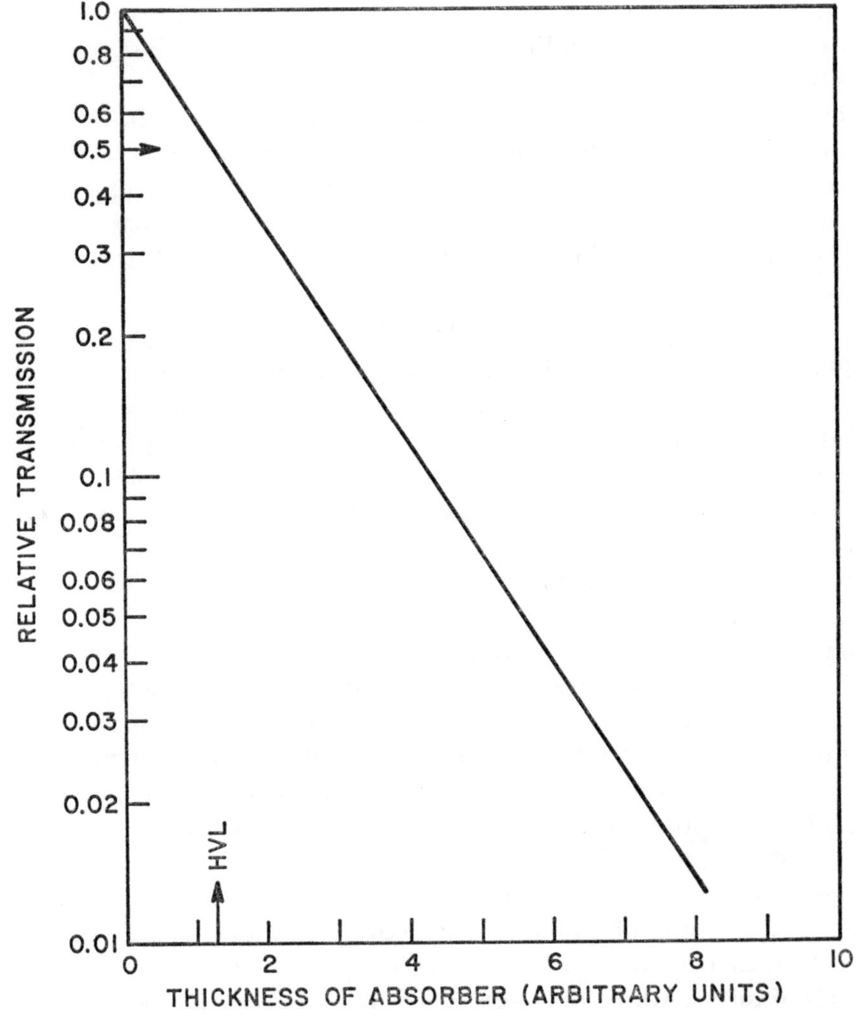


Figure 4-2. Exponential absorption of photons by matter. The slope of the line gives the attenuation coefficient.

interaction while 50 are absorbed. Sometimes it is convenient to work with HVL rather than with equation (4.5). By definition, $I/I_o = \frac{1}{2}$ when $X = $ HVL $= X_{\frac{1}{2}}$. Then equation (4.5) may be written as:

$$\frac{1}{2} = e^{-\mu X_{\frac{1}{2}}}.$$

Taking natural logarithm on both sides,

$$\ln\left(\tfrac{1}{2}\right) = \ln\left(e^{-\mu X_{\frac{1}{2}}}\right)$$
$$-0.693 = -\mu X_{\frac{1}{2}}$$
$$X_{\frac{1}{2}} = \frac{0.693}{\mu}. \tag{4.6}$$

The half-value layer can be calculated knowing the attenuation coefficient or vice versa. The attenuation coefficients for water and lead are shown in Figure 4-3.

> *Example 4.3:* The attenuation coefficients in water and lead for 140 keV photons from [99m]Tc are about 0.155 and 23 cm$^{-1}$ respectively. Calculate the HVL in water and lead for [99m]Tc photons.
>
> In water
>
> $$X_{\frac{1}{2}} = \frac{0.693}{0.155}\ \mathrm{cm} = 4.5\ \mathrm{cm}.$$
>
> In lead
>
> $$X_{\frac{1}{2}} = \frac{0.693}{23}\ \mathrm{cm} = 0.03\ \mathrm{cm}.$$

> *Example 4.4:* Calculate the fraction of 140 keV photons that will penetrate through 9 cm of soft tissue. Assuming soft tissue is water equivalent, then from the above example, 9 cm is two half-value layers. During the first 4.5 cm, 50 percent of the photons are absorbed and 50 percent are transmitted. Of the 50 percent transmitted, 50 percent are absorbed by the next 4.5 cm of tissue, resulting in a total transmission of only 25 percent.

> *Example 4.5:* Calculate the thickness of lead needed to transmit less than 1 percent of the photons from [99m]Tc.
>
> The transmitted photon fraction must be less than 0.01 or 1 percent. After one HVL the transmitted fraction is 0.5, or 50 percent; After two HVL the fraction is 0.25 or 25 percent; After three HVL the fraction is 0.125 or 12.5 percent; After four HVL the fraction is 0.0625 or 6.25 percent; After five HVL the fraction is 0.312 or 3.12 percent; After six HVL the fraction is 0.0156 or 1.56 percent; After seven HVL the fraction is 0.008 or .80 percent. Seven HVL reduces the photon fraction to 0.008 which is

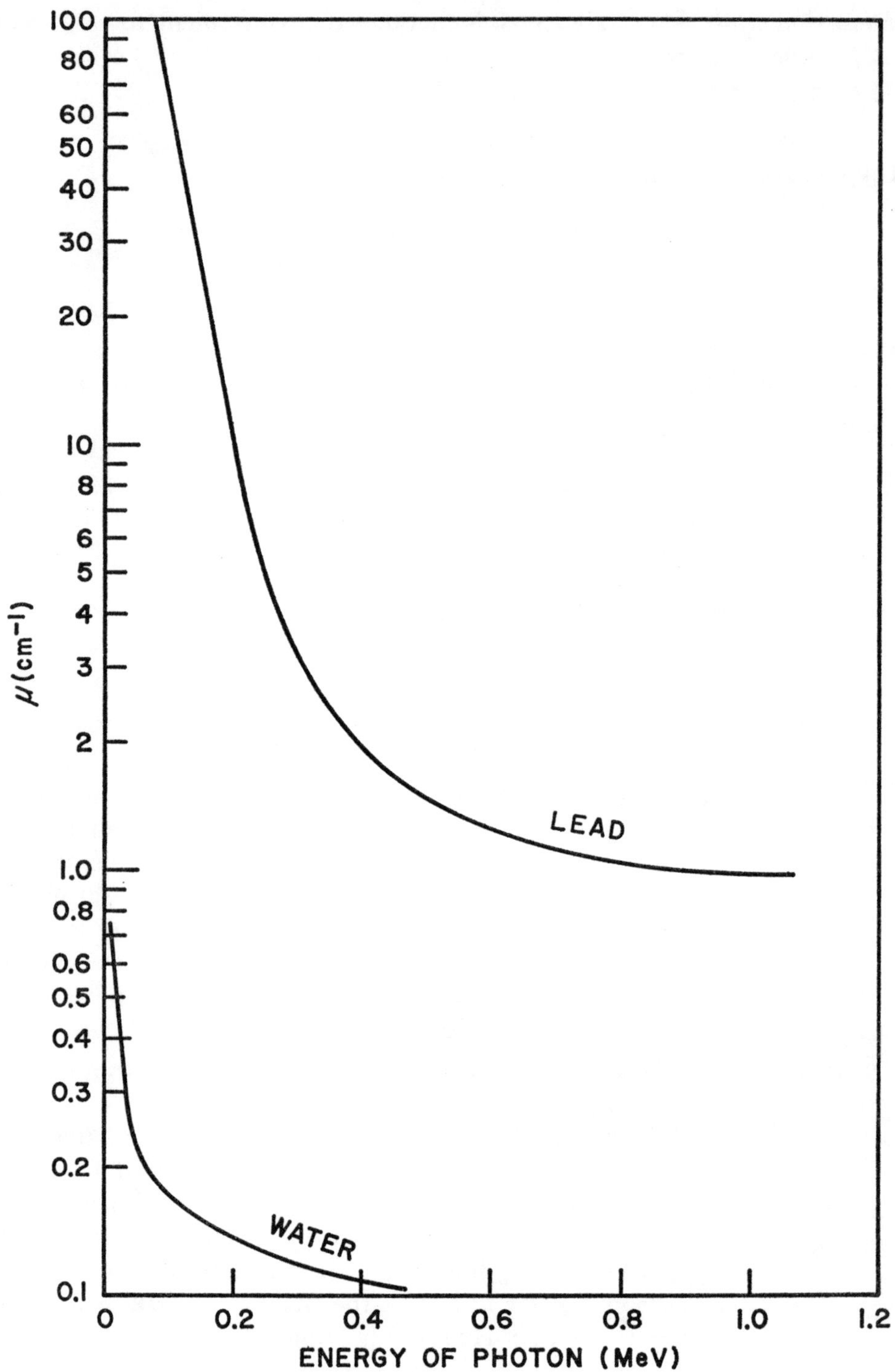


Figure 4-3. Photon absorption coefficients in water and lead.

less than 1 percent. HVL for 140 keV photons in lead from example 4.3 is 0.03 cm.

Thickness of lead needed $= 7 \times 0.03$ cm

$$= 0.21 \text{ cm.}$$

Another way to solve the problem is to use the formula

$$(\tfrac{1}{2})^n = f \tag{4.7}$$

where $n$ is the number of HVL and $f$ is the fraction of the photons transmitted.

This problem can also be solved by using equations (4.5) and (4.6).

Photons are much more penetrating than charged particles and have no definite range. The absorption process is more complicated than that of simple ionization. There are three processes that are mainly responsible for the absorption of photons:

1. photoelectric effect,
2. Compton effect,
3. pair production.

One or more of these processes may be responsible for the total absorption of the photon. The absorption coefficient $\mu$ which is the probability of interaction per unit distance is the sum of the probabilities of these individual processes. The energy of the photon as well as the nature of the absorbing material play important roles in deciding the dominant process of absorption. In order to develop suitable detectors for gamma-ray imaging it is very important to understand these processes.

PHOTOELECTRIC EFFECT. The electrons are bound in the atomic shells. The binding energy $B_e$ of electrons is different for each of the shells and increases with atomic number Z for a given shell. In some cases the energy $E_\gamma$ of the incident photon is completely given to a bound electron which is then ejected from the atom with a kinetic energy

$$T_e = E_\gamma - B_e. \tag{4.8}$$

This process, known as the photoelectric effect, illustrated in Figure 4-4, occurs mostly with the K electrons of the atoms of the absorber, provided the photon energy is greater than the K-shell binding energy. Characteristic x rays will be emitted as a result of vacancies in the K shell. The photoelectron produced, like beta particles, loses its energy as described before. When the photon energy is less than the binding energy of the K electron, an electron of a higher atomic shell such as *L or M,* whose binding energy is less than that of a K electron may be involved in this process.

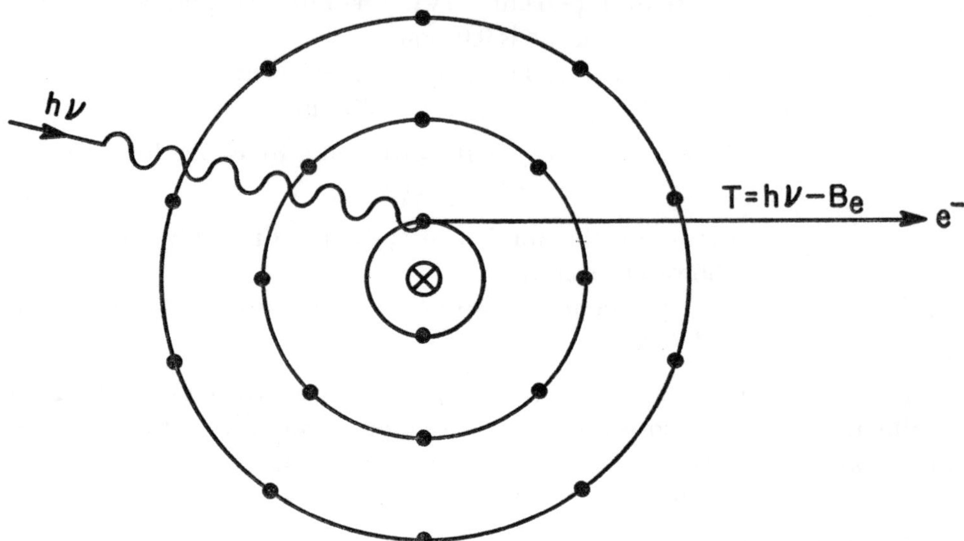


Figure 4-4. One of the bound electrons is ejected by the incident photon in the photo-electric process. The photon is completely absorbed by this single interaction.

*Example 4.6:* The K-electron binding energy of iodine is 33 keV. If a 140 keV photon undergoes a photoelectric interaction with a K electron of iodine, what is the kinetic energy carried by the electron?

$$T_e = 140 - 33 \text{ keV}$$
$$= 107 \text{ keV}$$

The photoelectric interaction is more likely to occur if the energy of the photon is just enough to knock out the electron. The probability decreases with increasing energy of the photon, approximately as $1/E_\gamma^3$ and increases with the atomic number approximately as $Z^3$. Therefore, for a given photon energy, the photoelectric effect is more important in heavy metal such as lead when compared to light metals such as aluminum. Similarly, for a given absorber, the probability is less for high-energy photons than for low-energy photons. This suggests that the photoelectric effect is mainly responsible for the absorption of low-energy photons by heavy elements.

COMPTON EFFECT. As the energy of the photon increases, the Compton effect becomes more important. In this process, the incoming photon knocks out an outer electron of the atom which is loosely bound. In doing so, it gives up part of its energy to that electron. The photon then moves in a different direction with reduced energy and increased wavelength. Because the binding energy of the outer electron is very small compared to the energy of the incident photon, the kinetic energy carried by the recoil electron is equal to

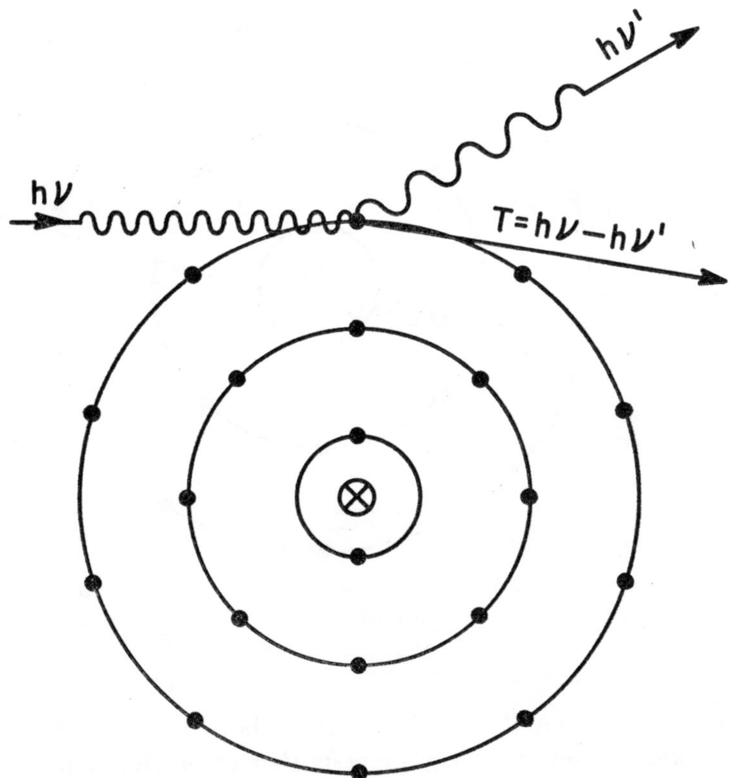



Figure 4-5. In the Compton process, the incident photon scatters with an outer electron, giving part of its energy to the electron. The scattered photon carries less than the original energy.

the difference of the incident photon and the scattered photon as shown in Figure 4-5. The photon is thus removed from its original path.

The energy of the scattered photon may not be the same for all Compton events; it depends upon the scattering angle. The fraction of energy given to the electron increases with the increasing energy of the incoming photon, and the energy of the recoil electron is lost by ionization as usual. The Compton process is inversely proportional to the energy of the photon and does not depend on Z since all elements contain about the same number of electrons per gram of matter.

PAIR PRODUCTION. When a high-energy photon passes close to the nucleus of the atom, it experiences the strong field of the nucleus. Then the photon may suddenly disappear, creating an electron and a positron. This is the inverse process of annihilation of an electron and its antiparticle positron. Mass is created from the energy as shown in Figure 4-6. The rest energy of an electron or a positron is 0.511 MeV. If the kinetic energy of the

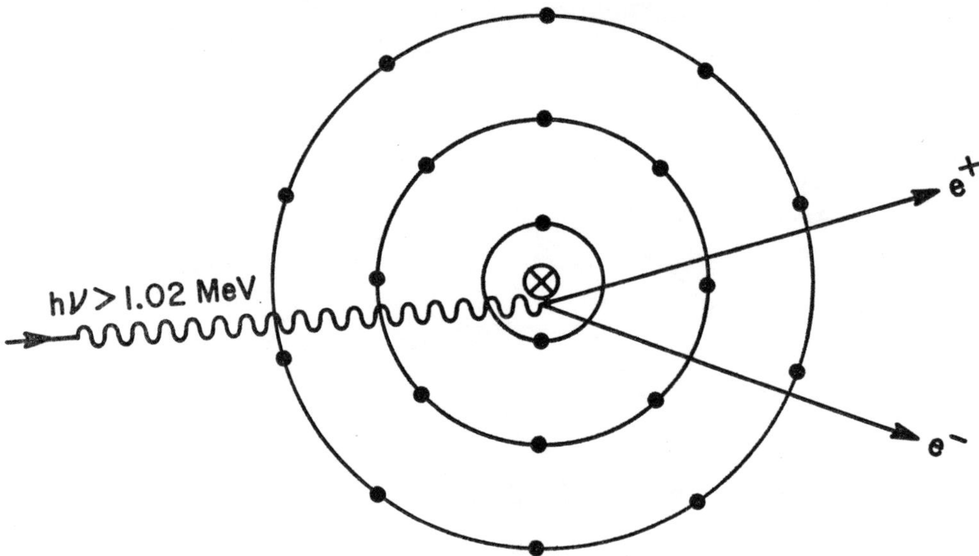


Figure 4-6. When a high-energy photon goes near the coulomb field of the nucleus, the photon disappears, creating an electron-positron pair. The threshold energy for pair production is 1.02 MeV.

created pair is zero, then the total energy of both particles is 1.022 MeV. The law of conservation of energy suggests that the incident photon energy must be at least 1.022 MeV to create a pair of beta particles. If the photon energy is more than 1.022 MeV, the remainder of the energy is shared by the pair.

$$E_\gamma = 1.022 + T_e{}^+ + T_e{}^- \tag{4.9}$$

where $T_e{}^+$ and $T_e{}^-$ are the kinetic energies of the positron and electron respectively. Pair production cannot occur if the energy of the photon is less than the *threshold* energy of 1.022 MeV. When this condition is satisfied, pair formation increases with increasing atomic number and increasing energy of the photon. Photons of energy greater than 1 MeV are of no use for radionuclide imaging in nuclear medicine, the reasons for which will be discussed in later chapters.

The processes most likely with different photon energies may be summarized as follows:

| | *Photoelectric* | *Compton* | *Pair* |
|---|---|---|---|
| Water (or soft tissue) | <0.05 MeV | 0.05 — 10 MeV | >10 MeV |
| Lead | <0.5  MeV | 0.5  —  5 MeV | > 5 MeV |

The manner in which photons interact with matter is a factor in the choice of radionuclides and appropriate instrumentation for imaging, which will be the subject of later chapters.

## PROBLEMS AND QUESTIONS

1. The range in air of an alpha particle whose kinetic energy is 4 *MeV* is
   - (A) 0.318 mm.
   - (B) 25 mm.
   - (C) 2.5 mm.
   - (D) 3.18 mm.

2. A radionuclide emits beta particles whose end-point energy is 1.5 MeV. The average *total* energy of the beta particle is about
   - (A) 1.5 MeV.
   - (B) 0.511 MeV.
   - (C) 1 MeV.
   - (D) 2 MeV.

3. The absorption of electrons from a radionuclide in matter is not
   - (A) dependent on the electron energy.
   - (B) dependent on the absorbing material.
   - (C) linear.
   - (D) exponential.

4. The approximate range of 1 MeV electrons in soft tissue is
   - (A) 3.9 mm.
   - (B) 0.39 mm.
   - (C) 0.55 mm.
   - (D) 0.16 mm.

5. The bremsstrahlung radiation loss by an electron of energy 5 MeV in lead is about
   - (A) 1.7 MeV.
   - (B) 0.7 MeV.
   - (C) 2.5 MeV.
   - (D) 0.08 MeV.

6. Positrons eventually annihilate with electrons in matter resulting in
   - (A) equivalent energy in the form of a photon.
   - (B) two photons of equal energy.
   - (C) two photons of equal energy in opposite directions.
   - (D) two photons in opposite directions.

7. The absorption coefficient for 364 keV photons of iodine 131 in tissue is about 0.1 cm$^{-1}$. The half-value layer is
   - (A) 7 cm.
   - (B) 0.05 cm.
   - (C) 3.5 cm.
   - (D) 0.1 cm.

8. The absorption coefficient for 364 keV photons in lead is about 1

cm$^{-1}$. The thickness of lead required to reduce the photons to less than 1 percent is

(A) 0.693 cm.

(B) 4.8 cm.

(C) 6.93 cm.

(D) 2.4 cm.

9. In the photoelectric interaction, the electron is ejected with an energy equal to

(A) the energy of the incident photon.

(B) the energy of the binding energy of the electron.

(C) the sum of the photon energy and the binding energy of the electron.

(D) the difference of the photon energy and the binding energy of the electron.

10. The absorption of 50 keV photons in iodine by photoelectric interaction is _____________ than the absorption of 140 keV photons

(A) much more

(B) slightly more

(C) less

(D) much less

11. A Compton-scattered photon in iodine is found to have 90 keV energy. The incident photons are from $^{99m}$Tc. The kinetic energy of the recoil electron is

(A) 140 keV.

(B) 33 keV.

(C) 50 keV.

(D) 90 keV.

12. The probability of Compton interaction

(A) increases with the energy of the photon.

(B) decreases with the energy as $1/E^3$.

(C) increases with the energy as $E^2$.

(D) decreases with the energy as $1/E$.

13. A 4 MeV photon disappears, creating a pair. The energy available to the particles is

(A) 4 MeV.

(B) 5.02 MeV.

(C) 2.98 MeV.

(D) 3.49 MeV.

14. In soft tissue, for $^{99m}$Tc photons, the important mode of interaction is

(A) photoelectric.

(B) Compton.

(C) pair production.

(D) all the above.

# 5

# Scintillation detectors

The detection of gamma radiation by any type of scintillation detector is basically a three-step process. A single gamma photon may interact with a scintillation crystal and produce light photons; the light photons transfer their energy to electrons inside a photomultiplier tube; and these electrons are collected and multiplied to form electrical pulses. The sequence is shown schematically in Figure 5-1. Each step will be discussed in more detail.

## SCINTILLATION CRYSTALS

A number of substances, particularly crystals, have the ability to absorb energy and reemit it as visible or near-visible radiation. The most widely used scintillator for gamma-ray detection in nuclear medicine is sodium iodide. Its advantages over other scintillating materials include (1) a relatively high density of 3.67, as well as a relatively high atomic number, thus increasing the probability of gamma-ray absorption, (2) a high efficiency, higher than any other solid crystals, for converting photon or charged particle energy to the energy of fluorescent radiation, (3) a transparency for its own radiation, so that large crystals can be used, (4) a short decay time for the fluorescent radiation (less than a microsecond), and (5) a fluores-

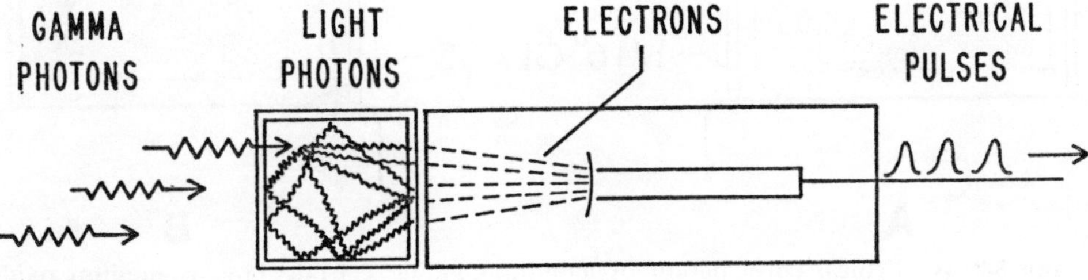


Figure 5-1. Schematic showing the sequence in the detection of gamma radiation by a scintillation detector.

cent radiation which matches the sensitivity of available photomultiplier tubes.

A sodium iodide crystal has a clear glass-like structure, and must be sealed in a light-proof and moisture-proof container. Part A on Figure 5-2 shows a small sodium iodide crystal, such as is used in a thyroid uptake probe. It is housed in an aluminum can with a reflective coating of magnesium oxide. A quartz glass plate allows the light photons to escape from the crystal and enter the photomultiplier tube. Part B on Figure 5-2 shows a crystal for a well counter. The hole in the crystal allows a test tube containing a radioactive substance to be placed near the center of the crystal, so that the probability is very high that any emitted gamma ray will be absorbed by the crystal.

Figure 5-3 shows the construction of a well counter. Since well counters are used for very small amounts of radioactivity, a large amount of lead shielding is required not only around the crystal but below it, to avoid scattered radiation and background radiation coming up through the photomultiplier tube. Thus, in any well counter the lead takes up more room than the rest of the apparatus inside.

## INTERACTIONS IN CRYSTALS

The production of light photons in a scintillation crystal is a complex one, shown schematically in Figure 5-4. An incoming x or gamma ray will interact with an electron in the crystal, by either a Compton or a photo-

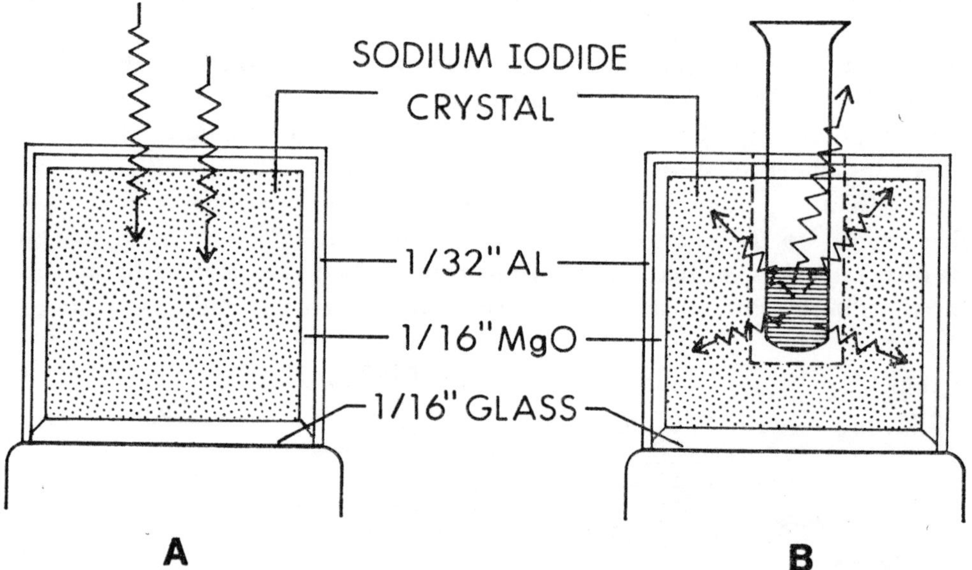


Figure 5-2. A. Typical construction of a sodium iodide crystal. The magnesium oxide serves to reflect light photons within the crystal. B. A well-type crystal.

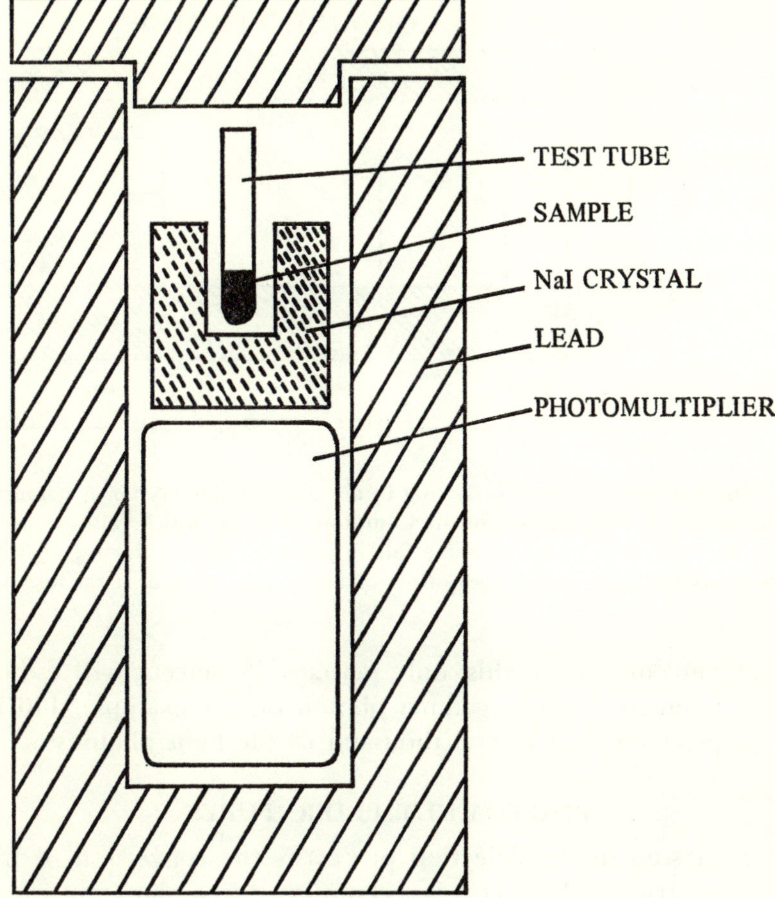



Figure 5-3. Construction of a well-type scintillation counter for counting samples containing small amounts of radioactivity.

electric process. This fast-moving electron will then interact with large numbers of electrons, producing ionization and excitation. These ionized and excited electrons may move to higher energy levels, known as the conduction band and the excitation band, until they fall into certain impurity centers, which act as energy traps. These traps are produced by the addition of certain impurities, called activators, into the crystal at the time of manufacture. For sodium iodide, small amounts of thallium produce the trapping centers, thus the nomenclature: "thallium-activated sodium iodide, NaI (Tl)." The trapping center may immediately give up its energy in the form of a light photon. In sodium iodide, the photons are centered at about 4050 Å, corresponding to an energy of about 3 eV per photon. Not all the absorbed energy reappears as light photons; for sodium iodide, the amount

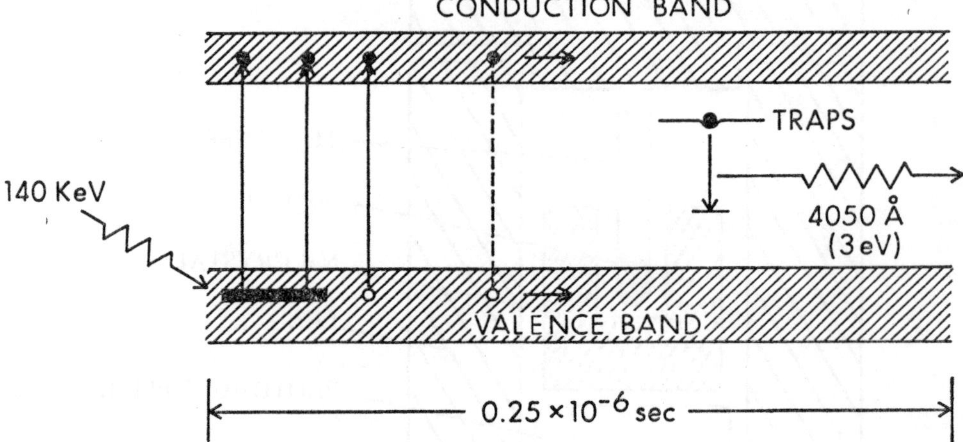


Figure 5-4. Diagram of the events occurring in a sodium iodide crystal. A gamma photon transfers its energy to a photoelectron or Compton electron, which raises large numbers of electrons to higher energy states. Some fall into energy traps, releasing light photons. The whole process occurs with a decay time of about a quarter of a microsecond.

is 10 or 12 percent, and of this, only perhaps 30 percent will escape from the crystal. Even so, a single gamma photon of, for example, 140 keV results in the production of several thousand usable light photons.

## PHOTOMULTIPLIER TUBES

The next step in the detection process is the conversion of the light energy into electrical pulses. This is accomplished in a photomultiplier tube. Figure 5-5 shows diagramatically the construction of a common type of photomultiplier tube. The inside surface, next to the crystal, is coated with a substance, such as an antimony-cesium compound, which easily emits electrons when struck by light photons. These photoelectrons are accelerated by a potential of several hundred volts between the emitting surface and the collecting surface, called the first dynode. Thus each electron striking the dynode releases five or more electrons which are accelerated and focused on the second dynode, and so on up to ten dynodes. The total gain of the photomultiplier depends on the voltage applied to the tube; typically this may be about a thousand volts, resulting in a gain of a million or more. Such a large number of electrons constitutes an electrical pulse, which may be counted directly by an electronic scaler.

Some electrons will be emitted spontaneously from the photocathode and the various dynode surfaces, resulting in noise pulses, which will gen-

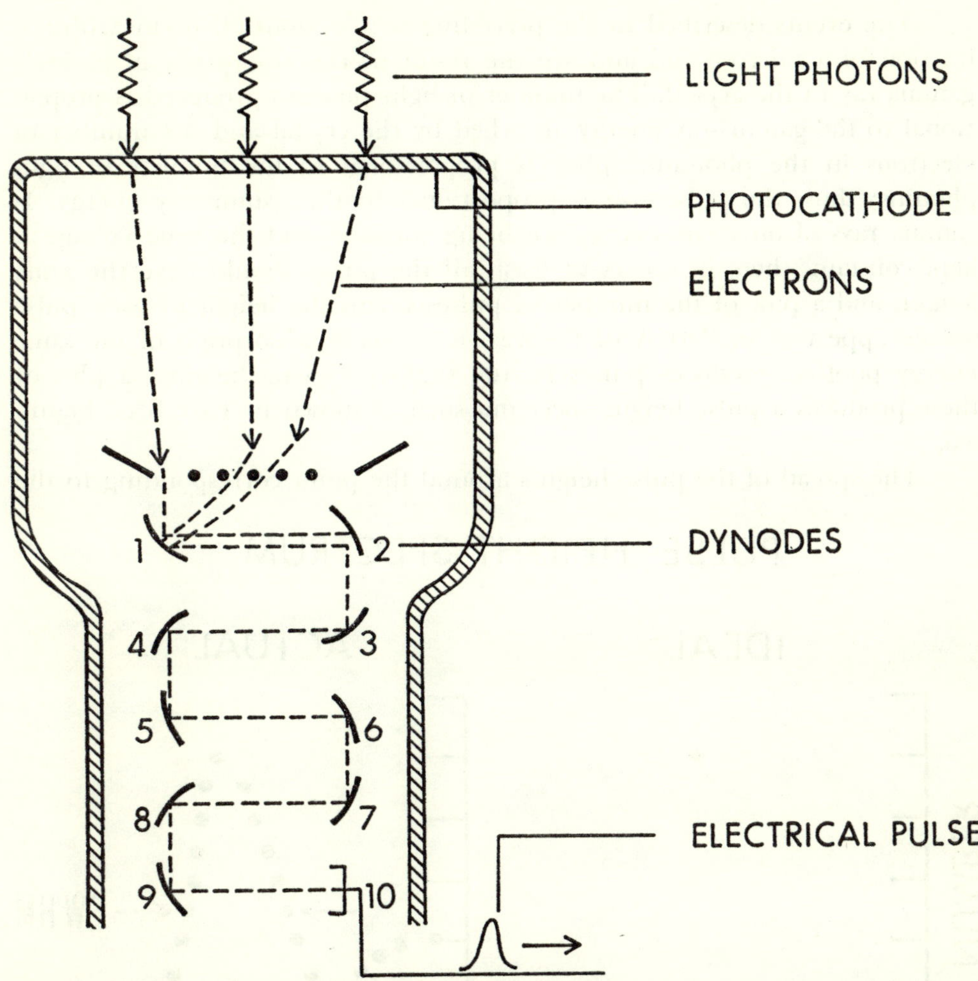



Figure 5-5. Construction of a photomultiplier tube having ten stages. Each electron striking a dynode may release five or more electrons, resulting in a total gain of a million or more.

erally be smaller than the pulses caused by photon absorption. Recent developments in photomultiplier design include the development of "bialkalide" tubes. These have photocathodes containing substances which have a greater sensitivity to the light photons from sodium iodide than does the antimony-cesium formerly used, thus resulting in an improved signal-to-noise ratio for the new tubes.

## THE PULSE HEIGHT SPECTRUM

The events described in the preceding two sections all occur within a fraction of a microsecond and are the result of the absorption of a single gamma ray in the crystal. The number of light photons produced is proportional to the gamma-ray energy absorbed by the crystal and the number of electrons in the photomultiplier is proportional to the number of light photons; thus, the pulse size is proportional to the gamma-ray energy. If gamma rays of only one energy are being counted, and the tube voltage is kept constant, then, in theory at least, all the pulses should have the same height, and a plot of the number of pulses versus the height of each pulse should appear as in Part A of Figure 5-6. Actually, absorption of the same energy photons produces pulses having slightly varying heights; a plot of these produces a pulse height spectrum such as shown in Part B of Figure 5-6.

The spread of the pulse heights around the point corresponding to the

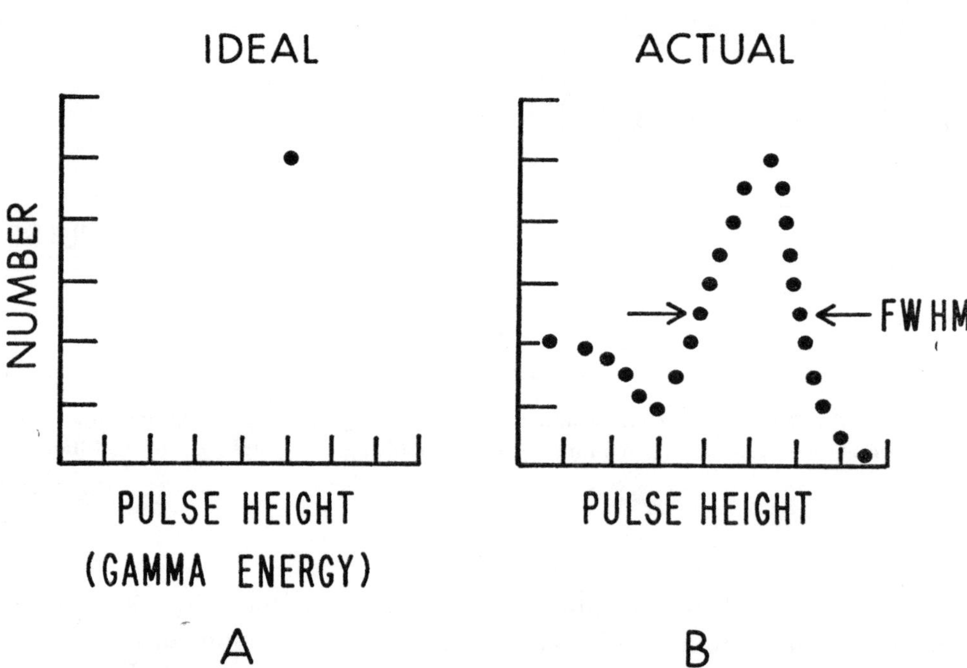


Figure 5-6. Plot of the pulses from a scintillation detector exposed to gamma rays of only one energy. The spread in the pulse heights may be described in terms of the width of the peak at half its maximum value, known as the full width at half maximum, FWHM.

gamma photon energy is caused, more or less equally, by three factors: (1) statistical variations in the number of light photons produced in the crystal by the total absorption of each gamma photon, (2) variations in the number of light photons reaching the photosensitive surface of the photomultiplier, and (3) fluctuations in the number of electrons released at each stage of the photomultiplier tube.

This spread in the pulse heights thus determines the energy resolution which the detector is capable of. The spread may be described by the term *full width at half maximum* (FWHM) which is the energy difference between the two points where the pulse height spectrum has half the height of the maximum point, as shown on Part B of Figure 5-6. The percent resolution is then the FWHM divided by the photon energy. For example, if in B of Figure 5-6 the peak corresponds to 662 keV and the half-maximum points are at 632 and 692 keV, then the resolution is $(692 - 632) \div 662 = 60 \div 662 = 0.09$, or 9 percent. The smaller the percentage, the better the resolution. The percentage energy resolution is dependent on the photon energy. For typical scintillation detectors it is about 8 to 10 percent at 662 keV, and about 20 percent at 140 keV.

The principle features of the pulse height spectrum from the scintillation detection of monochromatic gamma rays, and the events in the crystal which produce these features, are shown in Figure 5-7. These events may be briefly described as follows.

(1) THE PHOTOPEAK. These pulses represent the total absorption of the gamma ray energy by the crystal. The photopeak has a finite energy spread for the reasons just explained. The gamma ray may be absorbed in a single photoelectric process, or in a Compton process in which the scattered photon subsequently undergoes a photoelectric absorption within the crystal.

(2) THE COMPTON EDGE. A gamma photon may undergo a Compton process in which the scattered photon escapes from the crystal. In that case,

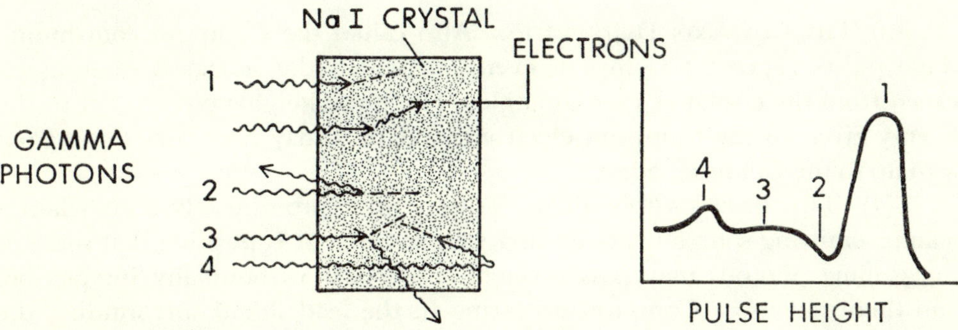


Figure 5-7. The principle features of a pulse height spectrum and the events in the crystal which give rise to them (see text).

the pulse height corresponds only to the energy absorbed by the Compton electron. In the Compton effect, the maximum transfer of energy to the electron occurs when the photon is scattered at 180 degrees, and the energy given to the electron is still less than the initial gamma energy by some finite amount, whose magnitude depends on the initial photon energy, as shown in Figure 5-8.

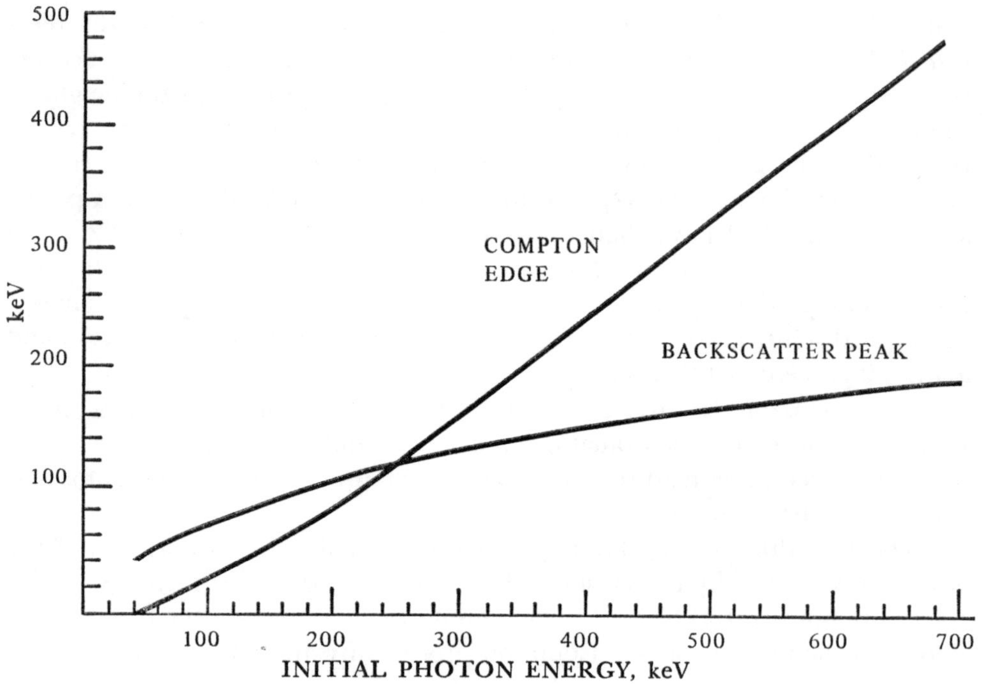


Figure 5-8. Plot showing the energy of the Compton edge and the energy of the backscatter peak as a function of the initial photon energy.

(3) THE COMPTON DISTRIBUTION. Also called the Compton continuum, these pulses represent Compton events in which the scattered photons escaped from the crystal at various angles. The pulse heights correspond to the energy given to the Compton electrons, and thus may have any value from zero up to the Compton edge.

(4) THE BACKSCATTER PEAK. This is most prominently seen when a gamma-emitting source is placed in a well counter. It is possible that some of the gamma photons may pass through the crystal without any interaction, and then undergo a Compton scattering in the lead shield surrounding the crystal (see Figure 5-3). If the scattered photon is given off at approximately 180 degrees, it may be detected by the crystal. If enough of such scattering occurs, a peak may be seen on top of the Compton distribution, at an

energy which depends on the primary gamma energy, as mentioned in Chapter 3, and also shown in Figure 5-8.

In addition to the above four features, other peaks may appear in the pulse height spectrum under certain conditions.

SUM PEAKS. When a nuclide which emits several gamma rays is being counted in a well counter, peaks will be seen which correspond to the sum of the gamma ray energies, and thus represent the simultaneous absorption of two or more gamma photons. Also, when counting a nuclide which decays by positron emission, peaks may be seen at 1.02 MeV, representing the absorption of both the 0.511 MeV photons produced when the positron unites with an electron. In addition, if the positron emitter also has gamma rays, peaks may be seen at $E_\gamma + 0.511$ MeV and at $E_\gamma + 1.02$ MeV.

THE IODINE ESCAPE PEAK. When counting low-energy gamma rays with a high-resolution system, a small peak may appear at about 28 keV below the photopeak. This occurs when an incoming photon knocks out the K-shell electron in an iodine atom, resulting in the production of a characteristic x ray. If this occurs near the edge of the crystal, so that the x ray escapes from the crystal without being detected, then the total energy seen by the crystal is less than the gamma energy by an amount equal to the K x-ray energy, which for iodine is about 28 keV.

Most of the above features are relatively minor issues; the real interest is in the pulses in the photopeak; these are the pulses which are normally counted, as their height is proportional to the gamma energy. However, when counting a radionuclide which emits gamma rays of several different energies, or when trying to determine the gamma spectrum of an unknown source, one must take into account all these features.

## DETECTION EFFICIENCY

The efficiency of a sodium iodide scintillation detector may be defined in several ways; furthermore, the same terms may be used to cover different definitions. However, two factors are of interest: (1) the fraction of the incident photons that will produce a scintillation in the crystal, and (2) the fraction of those scintillations that will result in a pulse corresponding to the photopeak, i.e. total absorption. The first factor is sometimes called the *intrinsic efficiency,* or the intrinsic total efficiency. It can be calculated, knowing the absorption coefficient for sodium iodide and the crystal thickness. The second factor is sometimes called the *photofraction,* and depends on crystal thickness, crystal diameter, and the geometry of the situation. The larger the crystal, the greater the probability that, in a Compton interaction, the scattered photon will be absorbed within the crystal. Thus a large-diameter crystal will have a higher photofraction than a small-diameter crystal of the same thickness.

The characteristic which is of most interest is the product of the above two factors, namely, what fraction of the incident photons will produce a pulse in the photopeak region. This is sometimes called the *intrinsic peak efficiency* and depends on crystal size, geometry and photon energy. Figure 5-9 shows the variation of peak efficiency with photon energy for several typical sodium iodide crystals.

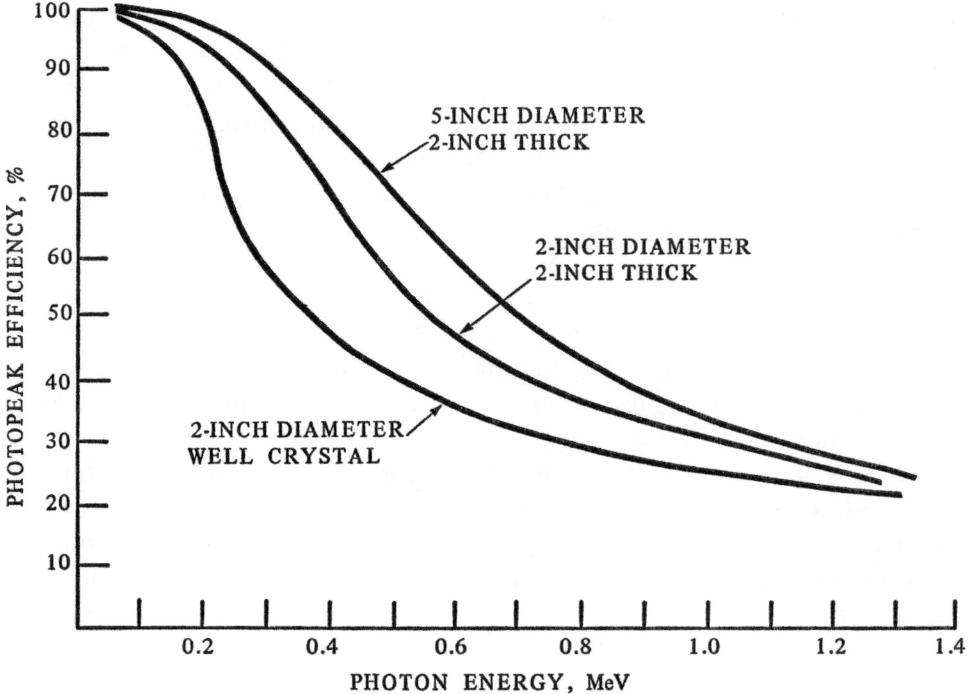


Figure 5-9. Plot of the photopeak efficiency, defined as the absorption efficiency times the photofraction, for several sizes of sodium iodide crystals.

## QUESTIONS

1. Sodium iodide is a good radiation detector because
   (A) it absorbs its own radiation.
   (B) it produces a large electric pulse.
   (C) it has a high conversion efficiency.
   (D) it has a long decay time.

2. A sodium iodide crystal
   (A) must be made of ultra-pure sodium iodide.
   (B) need not be hermetically sealed.
   (C) can only be made in small sizes.
   (D) has impurities added to produce trapping centers.

3. A sodium iodide crystal
   (A) produces one light photon for each gamma photon absorbed.
   (B) produces large numbers of light photons for each gamma photon.
   (C) converts all the gamma energy into light photons.
   (D) is not sensitive to beta particles.

4. A photomultiplier tube
   (A) multiplies the number of light photons.
   (B) produces one electrical pulse for each light photon.
   (C) produces one electrical pulse for each gamma photon absorbed in the crystal.
   (D) produces pulses which all have the same size.

5. If single-energy photons are totally absorbed in a crystal, the resulting pulses from the photomultiplier
   (A) will all be exactly the same size.
   (B) may have any size from zero to some value which depends on the energy.
   (C) will have a statistical spread about one value.
   (D) will form a continuous distribution.

6. In a pulse height spectrum from a scintillation detector the "Compton edge" represents
   (A) absorption of scattered photons in the crystal.
   (B) the maximum energy which may be given to a scattered electron.
   (C) a photon scattered 180 degrees and then absorbed.
   (D) the sum of all the scattered photons.

7. A large sodium iodide crystal
   (A) will totally absorb photons of any energy.
   (B) will not detect high energy photons.
   (C) will have an absorption efficiency which depends only on its thickness.
   (D) will be more efficient than a small crystal for medium-energy photons.

# 6

# Scanners

A scintillation detector mounted so that it could be mechanically moved in a raster fashion was the first widely used instrument for accurately mapping the distribution of a radionuclide in a patient. However, in recent years single-crystal scanners have been largely replaced by gamma cameras (which will be described in the next chapter). In most nuclear medicine departments, single-crystal scanners are now used mainly for obtaining high-resolution studies of the thyroid, while large dual-headed scanners may be used for bone studies and whole-body scans. In some cases, even the latter instruments are being superceded by scanning cameras, so that the role of the conventional scanner is becoming a very minor one. Nevertheless, a brief description of scanners will be given, since some of the principles to be discussed apply to gamma cameras as well as scanners.

## FOCUSED COLLIMATORS

In order to determine the distribution of radioactivity in an organ, the field of view of the crystal must be limited to a relatively small volume of tissue. The simplest construction for a collimator would be a single small hole in a block of lead; but this would be a very inefficient detector, so collimators normally contain many small holes, all pointing to or "focused" at the same point, usually about 6 or 8 cm in front of the face of the collimator. Figure 6-1 shows the cross section of a multihole-focused collimator. The spatial resolution will be greatest on a plane through the focal point, known as the focal plane. Both the spatial resolution and the relative spatial sensitivity of a multihole collimator can be shown by an isoresponse curve, which is a plot of the relative response of the detectors to a point source of

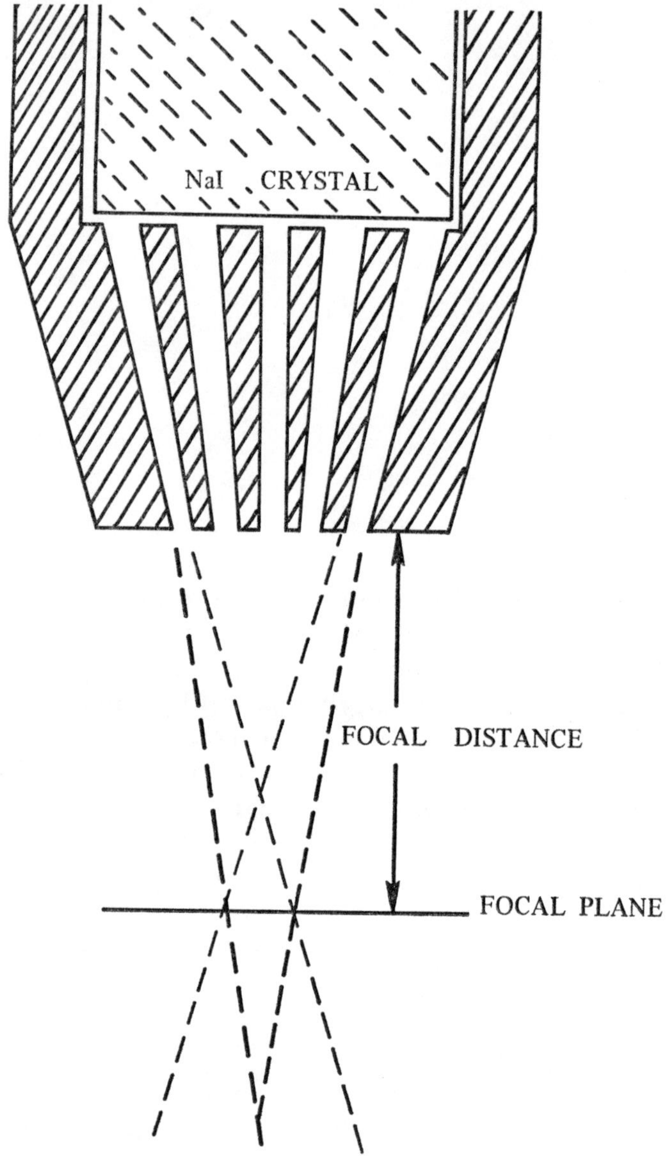


Figure 6-1. Cross section of a multihole-focused collimator.

radioactivity. Figure 6-2, Part A, shows a typical response curve in air, and 6-2, Part B, shows the response of the same collimator to a point source in tissue-equivalent material. Although in air the detector gives a lower counting rate for a source at the face than for one at the focal point, in tissue the attenuation decreases the counts coming from the focal region, resulting in a more uniform sensitivity with depth.

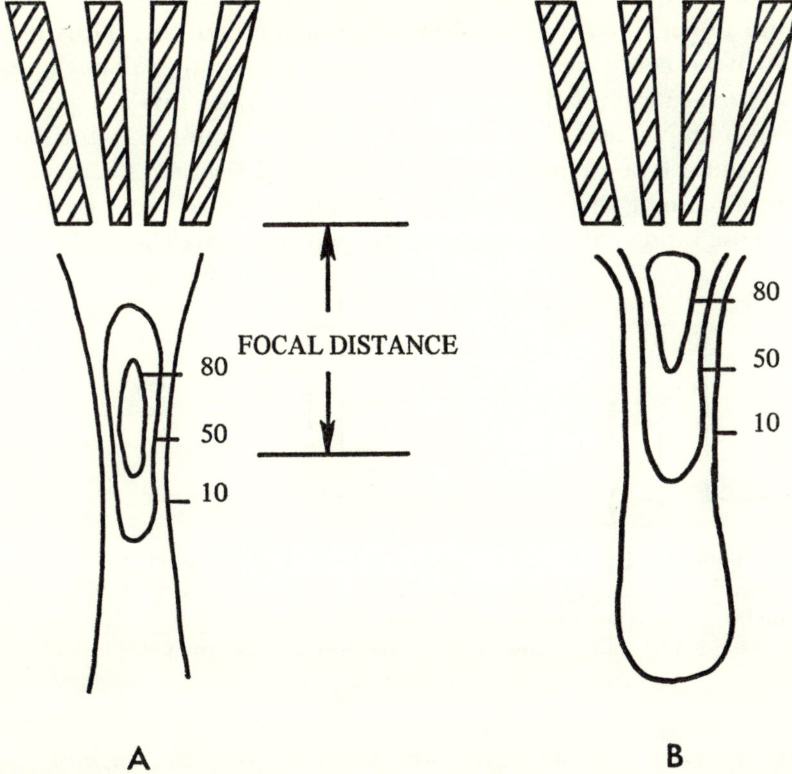



Figure 6-2. Isoresponse curves for a multihole focused collimator. A. Measured in air. B. Measured in tissue-equivalent plastic.

The spatial resolution of a focused collimator depends on the size of the holes; the smaller the holes, the better the resolution. However, for a fixed crystal size and a fixed septal thickness between holes, the more holes there are, the smaller the ratio of open space to lead, and thus the smaller the sensitivity. Collimator design is thus a compromise between good resolution and good sensitivity, complicated by the fact that the required septal thickness varies with the gamma energy. Ideally then, several collimators should be available for each gamma energy, depending on the user's requirements for resolution and sensitivity.

## PULSE HEIGHT ANALYZERS

Ideally a scanner should record only the radioactivity within the field of view of the collimator. However, when scanning a patient, some of the gamma rays from activity outside this region may be scattered by the tissue seen by the collimator, and thus produce counts in the detector. As discussed in

Chapter 4, a Compton-scattered photon will have less energy than a primary photon and so will produce a smaller pulse in the detector. Thus it may be possible to avoid counting scattered photons if pulses other than those of one particular size are excluded. The instrument for doing this is a pulse height analyzer, also known as a single-channel analyzer. Almost all scintillation detectors use some type of pulse analyzer. Figure 6-3 shows schematically the operation of a single-channel analyzer. Normally the window is adjusted so that only those pulses corresponding to the photopeak are counted.

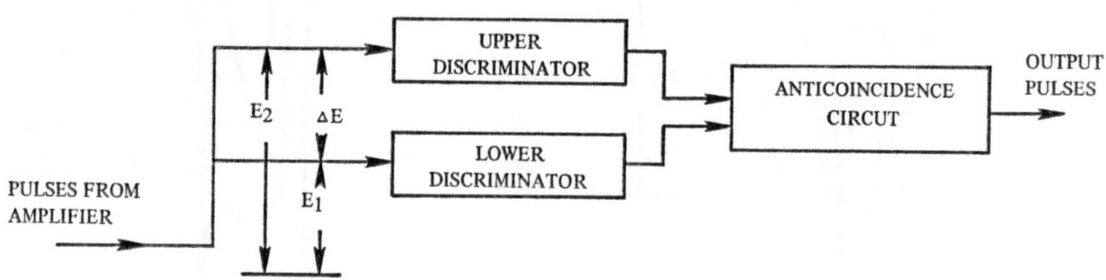


Figure 6-3. Schematic diagram of the operation of a single-channel pulse height analyzer. If the incoming pulse is greater than $E_1$, the lower discriminator puts out a pulse. If the incoming pulse is greater than $E_2$, both discriminators put out pulses. The anticoincidence circuit puts out a pulse when it receives a pulse from the lower discriminator only.

Some analyzers have separate controls for the baseline, or bottom of the window, $E_1$, and the top of the window, $E_2$. But a more common arrangement is to have a window width control, $\Delta E$, which is tied to the baseline. Then changing the "$E$" control in effect moves the baseline up and down the spectrum, while keeping the window width the same.

The size of the pulses reaching the analyzer may be changed in two ways: by changing the high voltage applied to the photomultiplier tube, and by changing the amount of amplification applied to the pulses after they leave the detector. It is convenient to vary one or both of these until the readings on the energy dials correspond numerically to the gamma energies in keV. This is known as calibrating the analyzer, and is best done with a gamma source having a single photon energy, such as $^{99m}$Tc or $^{137}$Cs. The appropriate methods for calibrating any particular analyzer are normally given in the manufacturer's instruction manual.

## READOUT DEVICES

The pulses from the analyzer are fed to a rate meter, which indicates the relative counting rate both by a meter and by an audible sound. Such a device is useful in locating the area to be scanned and determining the maximum count rate to be expected. The distribution of activity is most readily shown by the use of some form of tapper or printer which follows the motion of the detector and prints a line or symbol each time a certain number of counts have been received. Or the frequency of tapping may be determined from the rate meter, in which case it is possible to suppress the background, i.e. the tapper is only activated when the counting rate exceeds a certain pre-selected value. Mechanical printouts are useful in showing the distribution of activity while the scan is in progress. However, they will accommodate only a limited range of counting rates. As is the case with diagnostic radiographs, the blackening of a transparent type of film allows for a greater range of densities than does the blackening of a sheet of paper. Thus most scanners simultaneously produce a photoscan. A light source moves across an x-ray film in synchronism with the moving detector. The amount of film blackening corresponding to a given counting rate may be adjusted by varying the intensity or the duration of the light flash; thus a wide range of counting rates may be accommodated. Conversely, an adjustment may be made so that a small difference in counting rate covers a large range in film density, thus producing a form of contrast enhancement. In this way photoscans may be used as a simple means of performing a certain amount of data manipulation or image processing.

## WHOLE-BODY SCANNERS

For most general-purpose scanners, the area is limited to about the size of a 14-by-17-inch x-ray film. But the desire to do whole-body scans for bone tumor localization has led to the development of large-crystal scanners which can travel over the entire patient. The output of these scanners is not mechanically linked to the scanners. Instead, the detector position is sensed electrically and reproduced on a remote output device at any desired size; a reduction of five to one is convenient for total-body scans.

Obtaining a total-body scan in a reasonable time requires the use of a large crystal; in theory, the larger the better. However, practical limits are reached, both in the cost of the crystal, and in the weight of the lead required for shielding. Thus a five-inch crystal is about as large as can be conveniently and safely mounted above a patient and still move rapidly. Also, the use of too large a crystal with a focused collimator will result in poorer resolution for points above and below the focal plane, and thus may reduce the over-all resolution. One solution is to simultaneously scan the patient with two detectors, one above and the other below. Detectors with diameters as large as eight inches have been mounted under the table for whole-body scanning. Another solution is to scan the patient with an array of detectors. One such system uses ten adjacent crystals, each having its own focused collimator.

Although scanners are widely used for total-body studies, gamma cameras may also be used, either by taking multiple single views, or by the newer techniques of the "scanning camera," which will be described in the next chapter.

## TOMOGRAPHIC SCANNING

All large-crystal scanners are inherently somewhat tomographic. Since the resolution above and below the focal point is less than at the focal point, sources which lie above or below the focal plane will be less sharply imaged and thus to some extent blurred out. The magnitude of this effect depends on the angle of the outside collimator holes; the greater the maximum angle, the greater the tomographic effect. Thus with large crystal scanners, a certain amount of tomographic information can be obtained by taking several scans at different depths. However, this is time-consuming and not very satisfactory, and a number of instruments have been proposed or constructed for tomographic imaging. One of these is the two-detector tomographic scanner which is capable of transverse section scanning. Here the two opposing detectors make a series of scans at different angles around the patient, gradually building up a picture of the activity in the desired cross section. Such an instrument is mechanically very complex and few like it have been built.

One tomographic scanner which has become commercially available is the multiplane tomographic scanner developed by H. Anger and marketed by Searle as the Pho-Con®. However, this instrument uses two small gamma cameras as detectors and so will be described in Chapter 7.

## QUESTIONS

1. A multihole-focused collimator
   (A) focuses gamma rays onto the crystal.
   (B) is less efficient than a single small hole.
   (C) has all the holes aimed at about the same point.
   (D) cannot be used with a large crystal.

2. A multihole collimator which has good resolution
   (A) generally has low sensitivity.
   (B) also has good sensitivity.
   (C) has uniform sensitivity with depth.
   (D) has uniform resolution with depth.

3. The primary purpose of a single-channel pulse analyzer is
   (A) to avoid counting Compton electrons.
   (B) to increase the counting efficiency.
   (C) to avoid counting scattered gamma photons.
   (D) to decrease the counting rate.

4. Calibrating a pulse height analyzer refers to the process of
   (A) obtaining the maximum counting rate.
   (B) adjusting the pulse sizes to give the correct energy reading.
   (C) adjusting the window width.
   (D) obtaining the maximum pulse size.

5. A photoscan has an advantage over a paper print-out from a tapper because the photoscan
   (A) is faster.
   (B) is cheaper.
   (C) gives a more permanent record.
   (D) allows for a greater range of densities.

# 7

# Gamma cameras

A gamma camera was originally defined as a detector which remained stationary with respect to the patient and produced an image of the distribution of radioactivity in its field of view. Although recent developments have led to scanning cameras, the distinction between scanners and cameras still remains, in that a camera simultaneously collects information from a relatively large area of activity, whereas a scanner is sensitive to only one or at most a few points at a time.

## SINGLE-CRYSTAL CAMERAS

Most single-crystal cameras in use today are based on a principle first developed by Hal Anger around 1956. Figure 7-1 shows a cross-sectional diagram of a gamma camera. Normally a parallel-hole collimator containing thousands of small holes is used. A single sodium iodide crystal is used, in the form of a disk from nine to sixteen inches in diameter and approximately half an inch thick. The crystal is viewed by a large number of photomutiplier tubes; nineteen or thirty-seven are commonly used, although some cameras have as many as ninety-one!

The photomultiplier tubes cover a circular area slightly larger in diameter than the crystal and several inches above it. An optical light guide with beveled edges ensures that light which might normally fall between tubes is reflected into the nearest tube.

As mentioned in Chapter 5, a single gamma photon interacting with a scintillation crystal may produce several thousand light photons. All of the phototubes will receive some light photons, although the ones closest to the point of interaction will receive more light than those farther away.

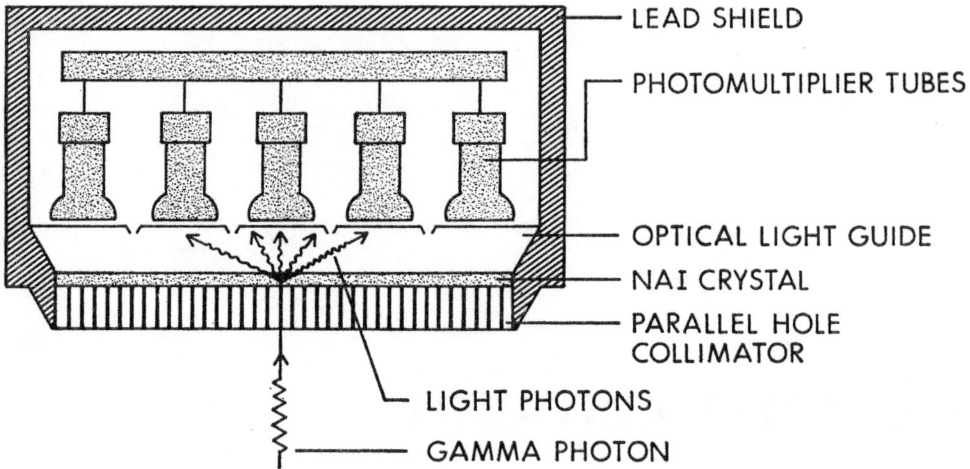


Figure 7-1. Cross-sectional diagram of a gamma camera.

The principle of operation is shown schematically in Figure 7-2. For simplicity, the crystal is shown with only four photomultiplier tubes. Now suppose a gamma ray is absorbed by the crystal at point "A." All of the photomultiplier tubes receive some light photons and send signals to the positional network. Here each tube's signals produce four pulses, called $+X$, $-X$, $+Y$, and $-Y$, which are weighted according to the position of each tube over the crystal, using the center of the crystal as the origin. Thus tube 1 produces a large $-X$ pulse and a small $+X$, a large $+Y$ and a small $-Y$. Tube 2 produces a $+X$ pulse which is larger than its $-X$ pulse, and a $+Y$ pulse larger than its $-Y$ pulse, although in this example all are smaller than the pulses from tube 1. Corresponding statements can be made about pulses from the other tubes. In the positional network all of the X pulses will be combined, and the Y pulses also combined to produce signals proportional to the $X$ and $Y$ coordinates of the event. These two signals are fed to the deflection plates of an oscilloscope. Meanwhile, the outputs of all the tubes are added together and fed to a single-channel analyzer. The total output is proportional to the gamma photon energy; thus if this pulse corresponds to the desired gamma photon, the oscilloscope is triggered, and a single dot appears on the face of the scope at a point corresponding to the point of interaction in the crystal.

Another method which has been used to obtain positional information makes use of delay lines. The output of each photomultiplier tube is connected to two delay lines, one for the X direction and one for the Y. The time of arrival of the pulses is then detected and used to develop the positional signals. Some improvement in the intrinsic resolution is claimed, al-

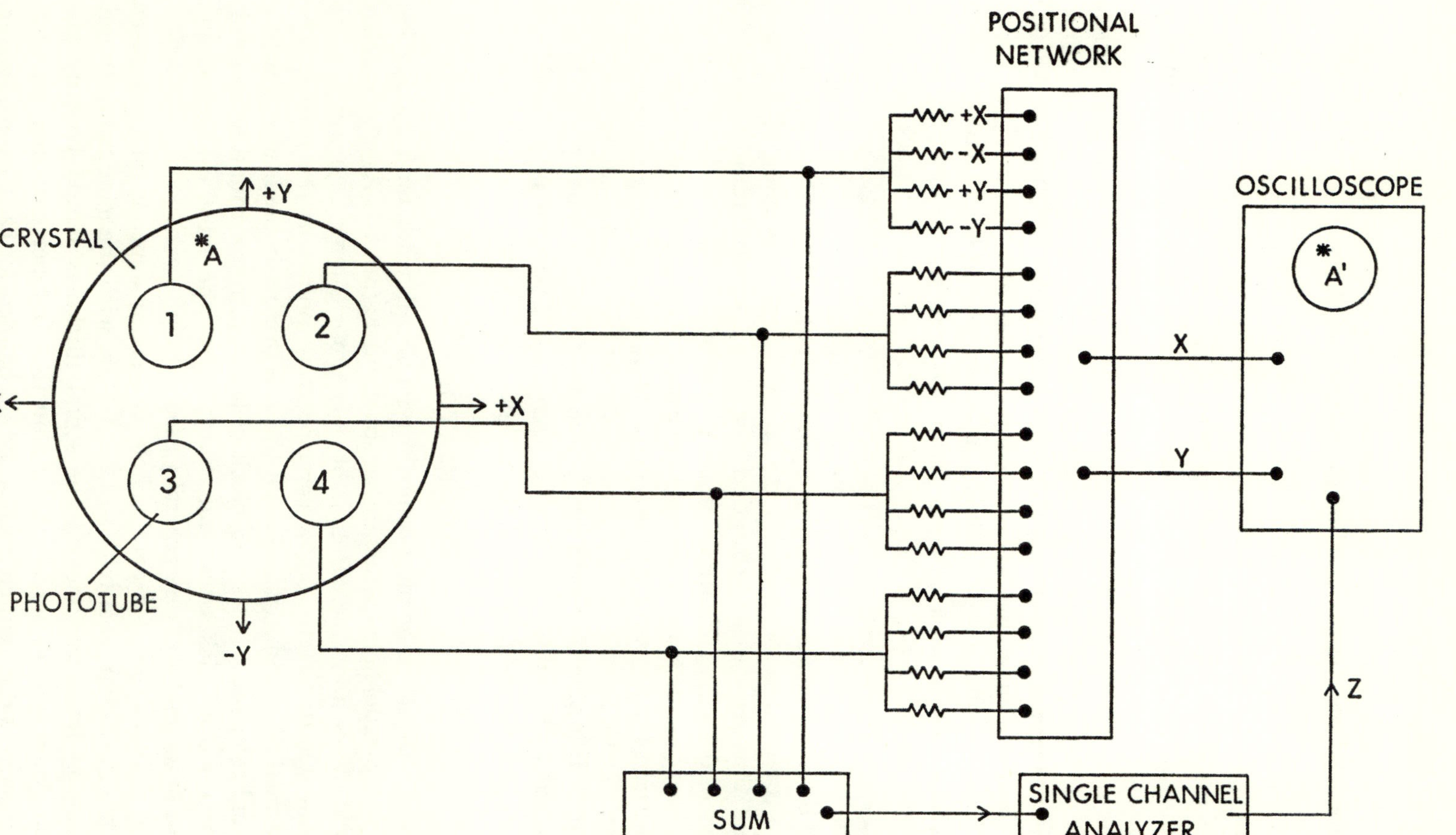


Figure 7-2. Schematic diagram to show the principle of operation of a gamma camera(see text).

though the actual resolution also depends on the stability of the photomultiplier tubes and the choice of collimator, as discussed later.

Another recent development has been the use of threshold preamplifiers on the phototubes. It was found that tubes which were far from an event did not contribute much toward localizing that event, because of random variations in the small signals from those tubes. Thus the use of preamplifiers which only amplify signals above a certain minimum value has resulted in some improvement in resolution.

The simplest way to obtain a picture is to place a photographic camera in front of the oscilloscope, open the shutter, and allow enough dots to accumulate; at least 50,000 are needed, although as many as 300,000 or 500,000 may be desirable sometimes, as discussed in Chapter 10.

The most popular type of photographic camera has been a Polaroid with three lenses, each set to a different f-stop. The production of three pictures thus gives a greater latitude than would result from a single black-and-white picture.

The suitability of the gamma camera for imaging with high-energy gamma rays is somewhat limited by the crystal thickness. The choice of one-half-inch is a compromise. Too thick a crystal would result in more light dispersion, and thus reduce the resolution; too thin a crystal would reduce the efficiency of detection. Figure 7-3 shows curves of the photopeak efficiency at photon energies for various crystal thicknesses. The photopeak efficiency is defined here as the percent of the gamma photons impinging on the crystal which will produce pulses corresponding to the full gamma energy and thus be counted. It is seen that for a one-half-inch crystal, photons up to 140 keV are counted with about 80 percent efficiency, and photons of 511 keV can still be imaged, although with less than 20 percent efficiency.

## COLLIMATORS

PARALLEL-HOLE. The most common type of collimator for a scintillation camera is a parallel-hole collimator, as shown in Figure 7-1. A large number of parallel holes allow penetration of only those gamma rays which originate from points directly below corresponding points in the crystal. The simplest method of construction, and the one originally used, was to drill a large number of small holes in a block of lead. However, round holes result in uneven septal thicknesses, and thus are not the most efficient shape; square or hexagonal holes are generally used.

The construction of a parallel-hole collimator depends on the desired compromise between sensitivity and resolution, with the gamma-ray energy also being an important factor. The septal thickness should be only just thick enough to reduce septal penetration to a few percent; thus for optimum efficiency, a different collimator should be used for each gamma energy.

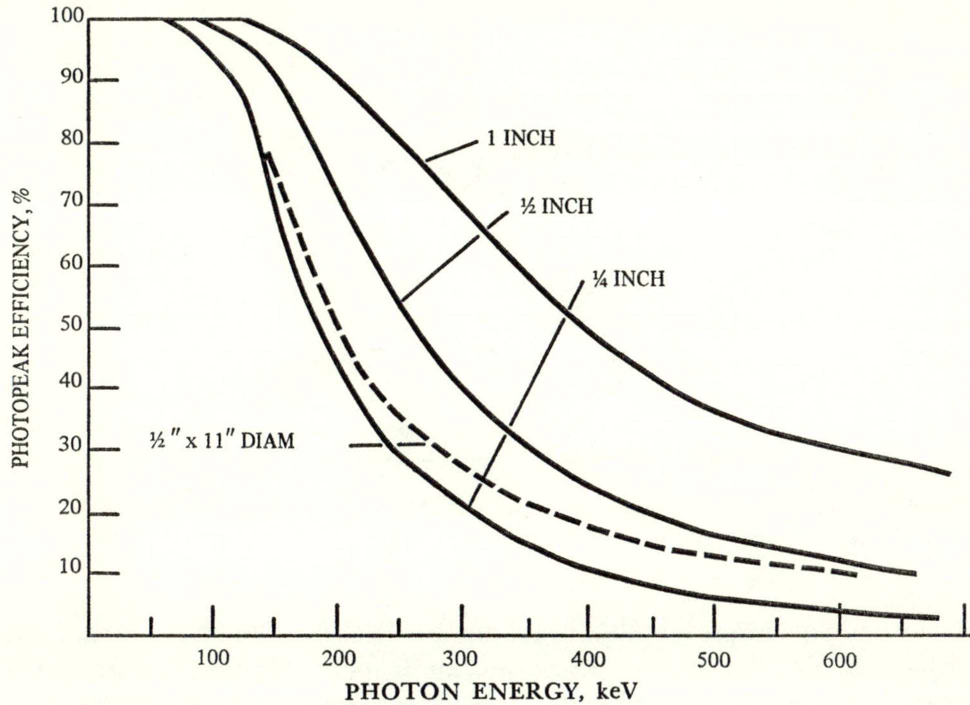



Figure 7-3. Solid lines: calculated photopeak efficiencies for three thicknesses of sodium iodide crystals.

Dashed line: measured values obtained by Anger (see the First reference in the section, "Additional Reading").

In practice, a "low-energy" collimator, designed for 140 keV, and a medium or high-energy one, designed for 365 keV, are all that are generally used.

For 140 keV photons from $^{99m}$Tc, the 5 percent transmission thickness is only about a millimeter of lead. Since photons must either pass obliquely through a septum or penetrate several septa before reaching the crystal, septal thicknesses of about 0.25 mm are commonly used. Thus a typical low-energy collimator may have 15,000 holes with a hole width of about 1.5 mm, septal thickness 0.25 mm, and height about 2.5 cm. The sensitivity may be increased in either of two ways: by increasing the size of the holes, and thus increasing the ratio of open space to lead, or by shortening the height of the collimator. Both methods results in a decrease in the resolution, both at the surface and at a depth, as discussed in the next section.

PINHOLE COLLIMATOR. A cross-sectional view of a pinhole collimator is shown in Figure 7-4. An enlarged view of the object is projected onto the crystal. The amount of magnification and to some extent the increase in

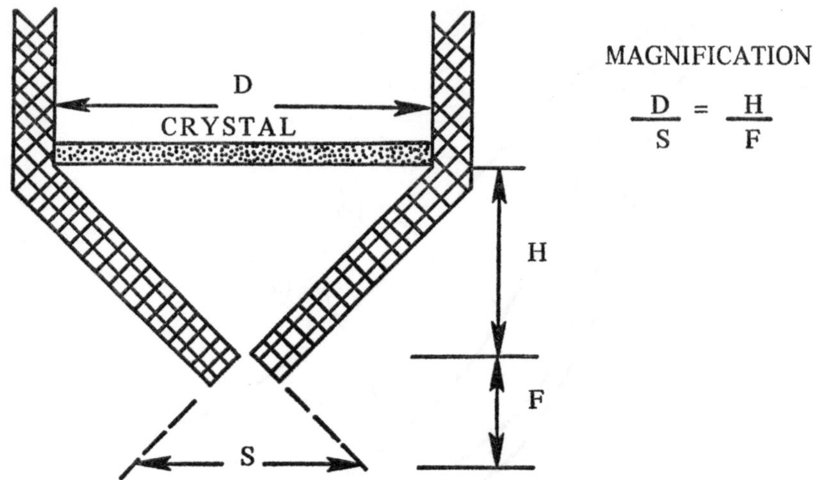


Figure 7-4. Cross section of a pinhole collimator. The magnification depends on the distance, F, of the source, S, from the pinhole.

resolution depend on the object-pinhole distance. The "pinhole" is not actually a pinhole, but may be 4 or 5 mm in diameter. Thus at high magnification the limiting factor in determining the resolution is the pinhole size.

The sensitivity of a pinhole collimator compared to a parallel-hole collimator depends on the pinhole-object distance. A small organ, such as the thyroid, may be imaged with counting times only slightly longer than those required when using a parallel-hole collimator, whereas an object as large as the crystal would require counting more than ten times as long. Thus the pinhole collimator is only useful for imaging areas appreciably smaller than the crystal size; but in such cases, the increased resolution obtainable makes it the collimator of choice.

OTHER COLLIMATORS. The converging collimator combines the advantages of both the pinhole and the parallel-hole collimators. Its construction is shown in Figure 7-5, Part A. Objects smaller than the crystal may be imaged somewhat magnified, thus increasing the apparent resolution while maintaining the high sensitivity of the parallel-hole collimator. The disadvantage is a decreased field of view. Also, there is some distortion near the edges of the picture, which is also true of the pinhole collimator.

Diverging collimators are also used, as shown in Figure 7-5, Part B. These are useful for imaging areas larger than the crystal, such as obtaining both lungs in a single picture. The disadvantage is the decreased resolution, as well as some distortion at the edges.

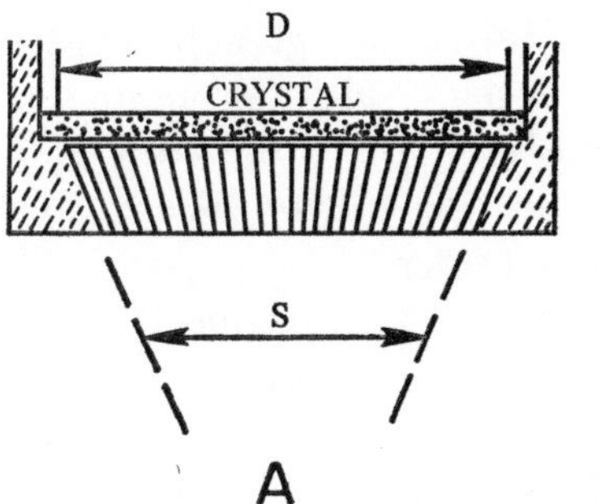 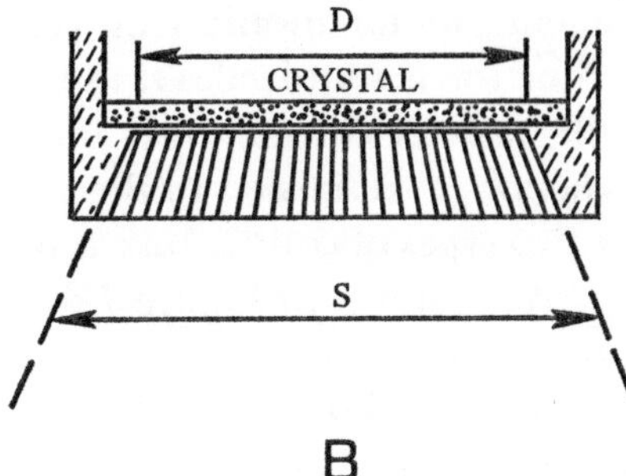

Figure 7-5. A. Converging collimator for imaging a source, S, somewhat smaller than the crystal diameter, D. B. Diverging collimator for imaging a source slightly larger than the crystal.

## CAMERA RESOLUTION

The ability of a gamma camera to accurately image sources of activity depends on a number of factors. These include the intrinsic resolution of the camera, the gamma-ray energy, the choice of collimator, and the distance from the collimator face to the source.

The term "intrinsic resolution" refers to the resolution measured without a collimator on the camera, which is an indication of the ability of the camera to distinguish between two closely spaced interactions in the crystal. The resolution may be measured in a number of ways. A simple and widely used method is the use of a bar pattern. This consists of a series of lead strips of various widths, separated by spaces equal in width to the adjacent bars. The intrinsic resolution of a camera may be measured by removing the collimator and placing a bar pattern directly against the crystal. A large uniform source of activity is then used (or a small source at several meters distance) and the width of the smallest bars which can just be resolved is taken as the intrinsic resolution.

In the range of 100 to 500 keV, the intrinsic resolution of a gamma camera increases, even though the sensitivity is dropping rapidly in this range. This increase in resolution occurs because those high-energy photons that are absorbed produce large numbers of light photons. Below about 75 keV, the resolution drops rapidly, since each gamma photon does not produce enough light photons for good positional information. However, since the most widely used nuclide is $^{99m}$Tc, most resolution comparisons are done using either the 140 keV gamma ray from $^{99m}$Tc, or the 122 keV gamma ray from cobalt 57, a nuclide whose long half-life and gamma energy make it useful for scintillation camera performance studies.

The measured intrinsic resolution is useful for comparing various cameras, or for monitoring camera performance; but to image a patient, a collimator is required. Of more practical interest is the resolution obtainable with various collimators. This resolution depends on the collimator construction, as discussed in the previous section. Figure 7-6 shows typical values for two types of collimators as measured on the same camera.

Also shown in Figure 7-6 is the effect of distance on resolution. The reason for this effect is diagrammed in Figure 7-7. Consider a point source of activity placed on the collimator face and centered on one hole (position 1). Then only the gamma rays which entered that hole would reach the crystal. As the source is moved away, adjacent holes begin to "see" the source (position 2). However, if the source is moved far enough away, the entire crystal will see the source, with complete loss of resolution. This emphasizes the importance of placing any organ to be imaged as close as possible to the collimator face, in order to obtain optimum resolution.

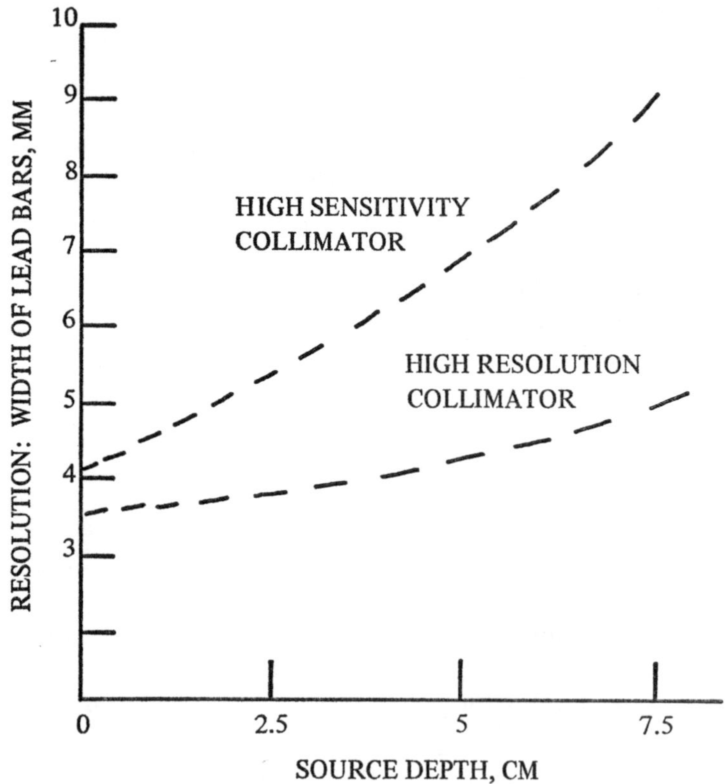


Figure 7-6. Resolution as determined by a bar pattern, measured at various depths in tissue-equivalent material.

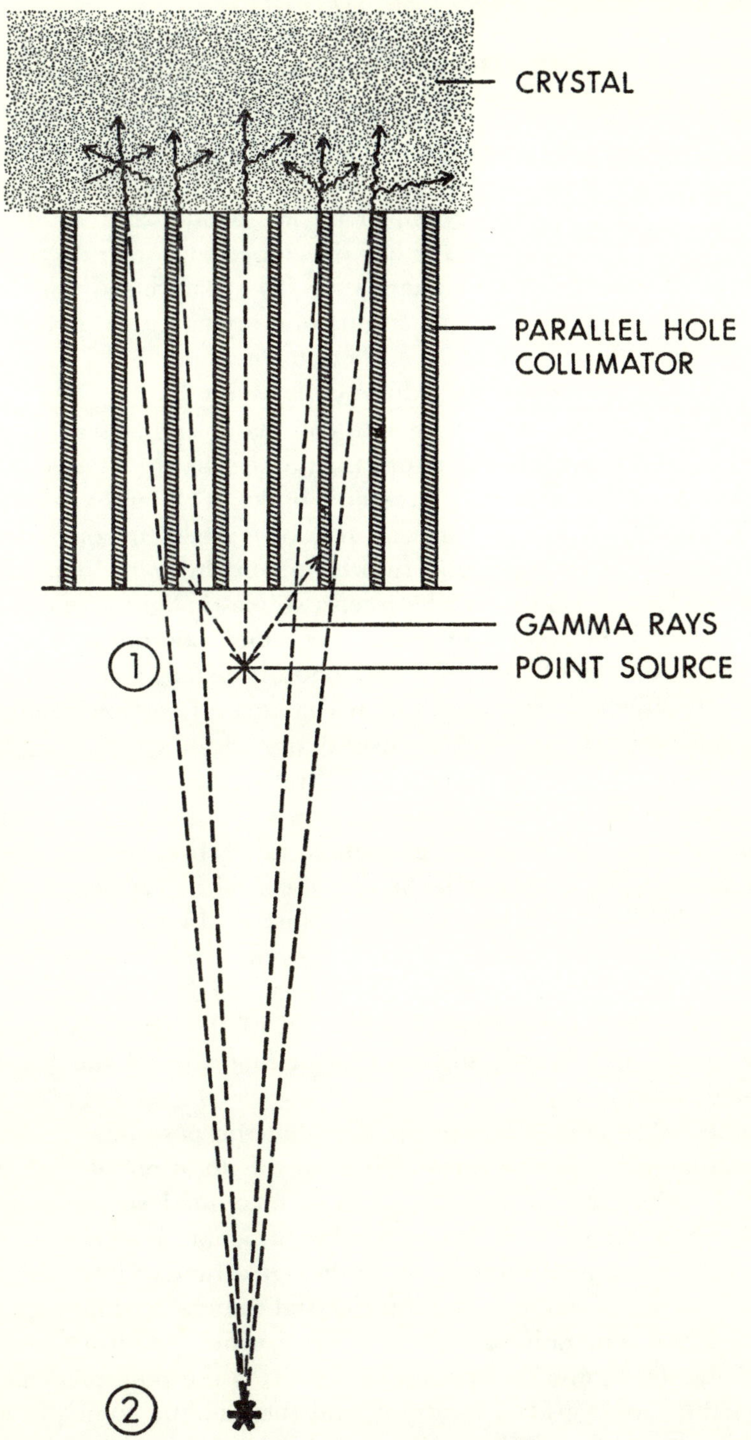


Figure 7-7. Enlarged scale drawing of a parallel-hole collimator showing the decreased resolution as a point source is moved away from the collimator face.

## THE MULTI CRYSTAL CAMERA

Single-crystal cameras of the type described in the first section are now made by a large number of manufacturers and widely used throughout the world. The second most widely used commercially available camera is the multicrystal type originally developed by M. Bender and M. Blau in the early 1960's, and subsequently further developed and manufactured by the Baird-Atomic Company. This camera uses 294 separate sodium iodide crystals arranged in fourteen rows of twenty-one crystals each, covering a field of view of about 6 to 9 inches. Each crystal is about 5/16 by 5/16 by $1\frac{1}{2}$ inches thick; the center-to-center distance is about 1.1 cm.

Each crystal has its own single-hole collimator and acts as an independent detector, as if it has its own phototube. Since the use of 294 photomultiplier tubes would be both expensive and bulky, a different arrangement is used. One phototube is used for each row of crystals and one for each column, requiring only fourteen plus twenty-one, or thirty-five phototubes. The light from each crystal is divided between two plastic light pipes, one leading to a "row" phototube and the other to a "column" phototube. The simultaneous detection of a light flash by a row phototube and a column phototube uniquely determines the crystal in which a gamma interaction occurs.

The multicrystal camera offers three major advantages over early versions of the single-crystal cameras, as well as several significant disadvantages. The use of crystals of $1\frac{1}{2}$-inch thickness results in somewhat higher counting efficiency for medium and high-energy gamma rays. However this advantage is not as great as it might appear to be. As discussed in Chapter 4, photons of more than a few hundred keV interact primarily by the Compton process. Since the single crystals are only 7/16 inches on a side, the probability that the scattered photon will escape from the crystal is quite high. Thus the photopeak efficiency, the probability that all of the photon energy will be absorbed in a crystal, is only slightly greater than that of the $\frac{1}{2}$-by-9-inch-diameter single crystal.

Another advantage is due to the fact that the positional information is already available in digital form. That is, the location of each crystal is known and the number of interactions in each counted, so that data manipulation can be performed, i.e. background subtraction, counts per unit time, comparison of regions of interest, and other quantitative information. However, since the introduction of the multicrystal camera, various accessories for the single-crystal camera have been developed which perform the same functions. Briefly, the accessories operate by digitizing the positional information signals, establishing a grid of locations, and then adding counts to each location as they are produced. Thus the same kinds of quantitative information can now be obtained with either type of camera.

A third advantage of the multicrystal camera is its ability to handle higher counting rates, at least compared to earlier versions of the single-crystal camera. Since each crystal acts as an independent detector, the time required to determine the positional coordinates of an event is less. The use of fast electronics has resulted in dead times of only about 2 $\mu$sec (microseconds), compared to times of 5 to 10 $\mu$sec typical of single-crystal cameras. However, recently improvements in single-crystal cameras have resulted in several models now having dead times of only a few microseconds, thus largely matching the high count rate performance formerly available only with the multicrystal camera.

One disadvantage of the multicrystal camera is the poor energy resolution, which is the result of loss of light photons in the light pipes which lead from the crystals to the phototubes. The energy resolution is a function of gamma photon energy, but at 140 keV the resolution is about 50 percent, compared with 15 percent to 20 percent for single-crystal cameras. This makes it difficult to exclude scattered photons by pulse height analysis.

A major disadvantage inherent in earlier versions of the multicrystal camera was the spatial resolution. Since the crystal spacing is about 1.1 cm, the resolution cannot be measured in the usual sense, that is, by the resolution of a bar pattern, since two line sources can only be resolved if they are more than 2 cm apart, so that there is a dark crystal between them. However, the resolution problem has been solved, at least for static studies, by recent introduction of the multiposition measurement technique. Since the crystals have tapered collimator holes with the narrow end at the face of the collimator, the field of view of each crystal is less than the crystal size. Thus there is some advantage to taking views between crystal centers, so to speak. This is accomplished by moving the source to sixteen different positions within a 1.1 by 1.1 cm square and recording counts for equal times at each position. The resulting picture has a resolution comparable to that obtainable with a single-crystal camera.

## TOMOGRAPHIC CAMERAS

The output of most gamma cameras and scanners is, like a radiograph, a two-dimensional picture of three-dimensional structures. Some information about the depth of these structures can be obtained by taking multiple views from different directions, as is sometimes done in radiography. However, such procedures are time consuming and often present difficulties in positioning the camera and patient. Hence there is need for a camera which can obtain tomographic information without repositioning the patient.

Two types of tomographic apparatus which are commercially available are the tomocamera attachment available as an accessory on the Searle (formerly Nuclear-Chicago) cameras, and the tomoscanner, developed by H. Anger and marketed by Searle as the Pho-Con. The tomocamera operates on a principle somewhat similar to that used to produce tomographic radiographs. In x-ray tomography, the tube above the patient and the film below the patient move in opposite directions during the exposure. The result is that only those objects which lie in a horizontal plane containing the axis of rotation are in focus; objects above and below this plane are blurred out. In the tomocamera, the camera itself remains stationary, but the collimator, which is a parallel-hole type in which all the holes are slanted at a slight angle, rotates 360 degrees about a vertical axis during the exposure. Meanwhile the patient is mechanically moved—not rotated, but rather translated in a small circular path—so that the central hole of the collimator always aims at the same point in the patient, which is in the mechanical focal plane. The camera picture will thus image only those sources which lie in the focal plane, while those above and below are blurred out. Correction signals which vary with the degree of rotation are then added to the positional information signals so that the location of sources above and below the focal plane can be determined. Thus multiple tomographic views can be obtained from a single rotation.

The tomocamera and similar rotating devices suffer from the same trouble as x-ray tomography, namely artifacts, in this case circular artifacts from sources which lie above or below the plane of interest. This type of difficulty is largely overcome by the use of a different principle in the Pho-Con multiplane tomographic scanner. This apparatus contains two small gamma cameras, one above the patient and one below, which scan the patient in the same manner as a dual-probe whole-body scanner. Each camera has a single crystal, 8 inches in diameter and $1\frac{1}{2}$ inches thick, viewed by seven phototubes, and uses a focused collimator. The method of producing tomograms may be illustrated by considering only one camera and two point sources at different distances from the face of the collimator, as shown in Figure 7-8. As the camera moves, the position of the sources with respect to the camera changes; consider three locations, 1, 2, and 3. The picture seen on the cathode ray tube is then shown at the three corresponding times; source *A* appears as a moving dot, while source *B* is only seen when at location 2, at which time it nearly fills the camera. The image seen on the cathode ray tube is projected onto a moving film, which moves in synchronism with the camera, using a different lens system for each plane of interest. Each lens system has a different magnification and projects its image onto a different part of the moving film. The first lens system projects a slightly reduced image, so that point *A* appears stationary with respect to the moving film; the lens system for *B* projects a greatly reduced image onto the moving film. Thus for points near the geometric focus, the camera system acts like

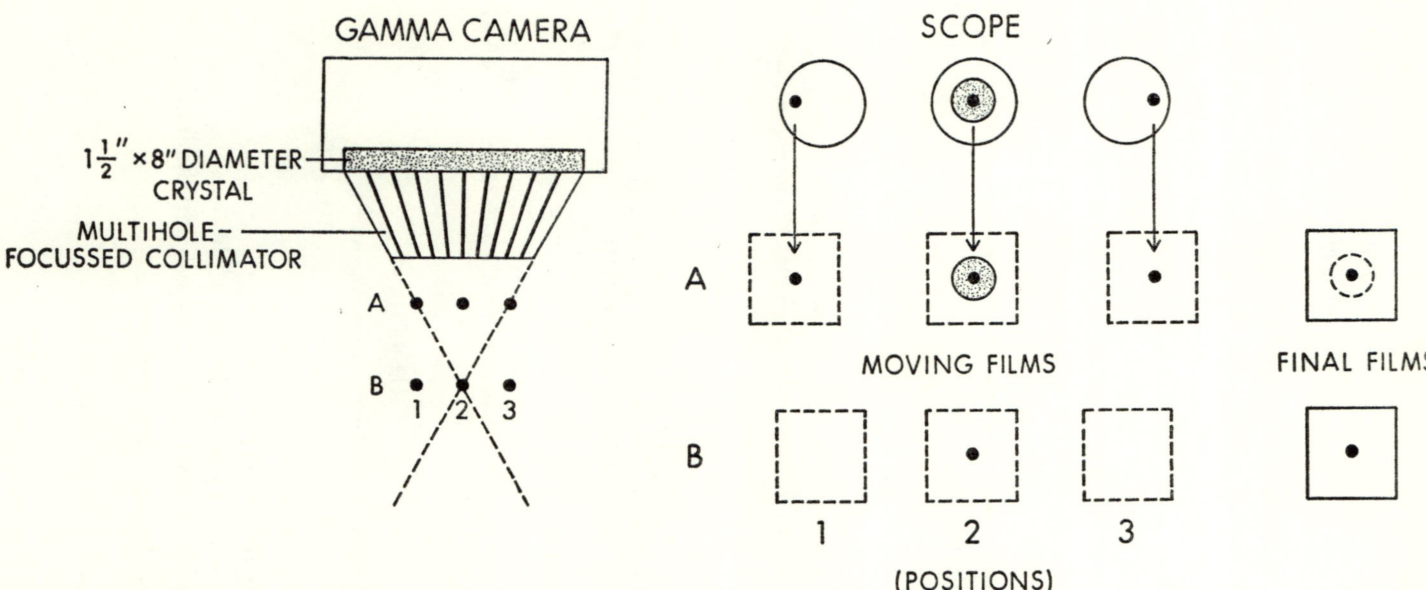



Figure 7-8. Simplified diagram of the operation of the multiplane tomographic scanner (see text). Adapted from Anger (see the third reference in the section, "Additional Reading."

the conventional single-crystal scanner. For points below the geometric focus, the lens systems invert the image of the cathode ray tube. By using six lens systems, points at six different depths may be imaged on different areas of the moving film, resulting in the simultaneous production of six tomographic pictures.

Each detected gamma ray produces a dot on all six films; however, the lens systems cause the dots to appear in such a manner that only structures at a given depth are in focus on the tomogram corresponding to that depth. Dots from other depths are evenly dispersed over a disk-shaped area, thus minimizing the production of artifacts caused by false summations.

In addition to producing tomograms, the multiplane tomographic scanner offers better resolution than the conventional scanner at all depths except at the focal plane, where the resolution of the two types is comparable. Also, the use of larger detectors results in greater sensitivity and, as a result, improved counting statistics.

## ADDITIONAL READING

### *Single-Crystal Cameras*

Anger, H. O.: Sensitivity and resolution of the scintillation camera. In Gottschalk, A., and Beck, R. N., (Eds.): *Fundamental Problems in Scanning*. Springfield, Thomas, 1968.

### *Multicrystal Cameras*

Grenier, R. P., Bender, M. A., and Jones, R. H.: A computerized multi-crystal scintillation camera. In Hine, G. J., and Sorenson, J. A. (Eds.): *Instrumentation in Nuclear Medicine*. New York, Academic Press, 1974, Vol. II.

### *Tomographic Cameras*

Anger, H. O.: Tomography and other depth-discrimination techniques. In Hine, G. J., and Sorenson, J. A., (Eds.): *Instrumention in Nuclear Medicine*. New York, Academic Press, 1974, Vol. II.

## QUESTIONS

1. The advantages of a gamma camera over a scanner include which of the following:
   (1) better resolution,
   (2) greater sensitivity,
   (3) greater efficiency for high-energy photons,
   (4) more uniform resolution and sensitivity with depth,
   (5) ability to do dynamic studies.
     (A) 1,2
     (B) 2,3,4
     (C) 1,4,5
     (D) 2,5

2. In general, for a parallel-hole collimator, the more holes there are,
    (A) the greater the sensitivity.
    (B) the greater the resolution.
    (C) the better it is for high-energy photons.
    (D) the thicker it has to be.

3. Which of the following collimators can provide an enlarged image:
    (1) parallel hole.
    (2) diverging.
    (3) converging.
    (4) pinhole.
        (A) 1,2
        (B) 3,4
        (C) 1,3
        (D) 1,2,3,4

4. The spatial resolution of a gamma camera is
    (A) greatest at the focal plane.
    (B) greatest at the face of the collimator.
    (C) uniform with depth.
    (D) independent of the collimator thickness.

5. The spatial resolution of a gamma camera
    (A) is greatest for low-energy photons.
    (B) does not vary with photon energy.
    (C) is greater for high-energy photons.
    (D) is proportional to the efficiency of detection.

6. The advantages of the multicrystal camera over most single-crystal cameras include
    (1) better spatial resolution.
    (2) higher counting rates.
    (3) greater efficiency for high-energy photons.
    (4) better energy resolution.
    (5) larger field of view.
        (A) 1,2,3
        (B) 2,3
        (C) 1,3,5
        (D) 3,4

7. Most tomographic gamma cameras
    (A) require a separate exposure for each plane of interest.
    (B) cannot be used for static imaging.
    (C) produce some artifacts and ghost images.
    (D) give poor spatial resolution.

# 8

# Other imaging devices

## POSITRON CAMERAS

As mentioned in the previous chapters, a free positron eventually annihilates with an electron resulting in the production of two photons of energy 511 keV emitted in the opposite directions. These photons can be effectively used to obtain the distribution pattern of a positron-emitting radionuclide administered to a patient. A good example is fluorine-18, which is useful for skeletal scanning. However, in scanning with $^{18}$F, only one of the two simultaneously emitted 511 keV photons is normally used to obtain the image.

The emission of two annihilation gamma rays precisely related in time and direction allows coincidence detection with a positron camera. The basic principle is to use two scintillation detectors placed on opposite sides of a radiation source as shown in Fig 8-1. Each detector is equipped with the usual amplifier and energy discriminator. The output from the energy discriminators is then fed to a *coincidence unit* which will give an output pulse only when the events from the detectors are separated by less than the resolving time of the coincidence unit which is usually of the order of a tenth of a microsecond. In other words, the purpose of the coincidence unit is to accept input pulses arriving almost simultaneously in time and reject all others. The output pulses from the coincidence unit can then be used to obtain the image.

The counts obtained with a positron camera are the sum of "true" coincidence and "chance" coincidence counts. The event (a) shown in Figure 8-1 will be counted as a true coincidence count, while the events (b)

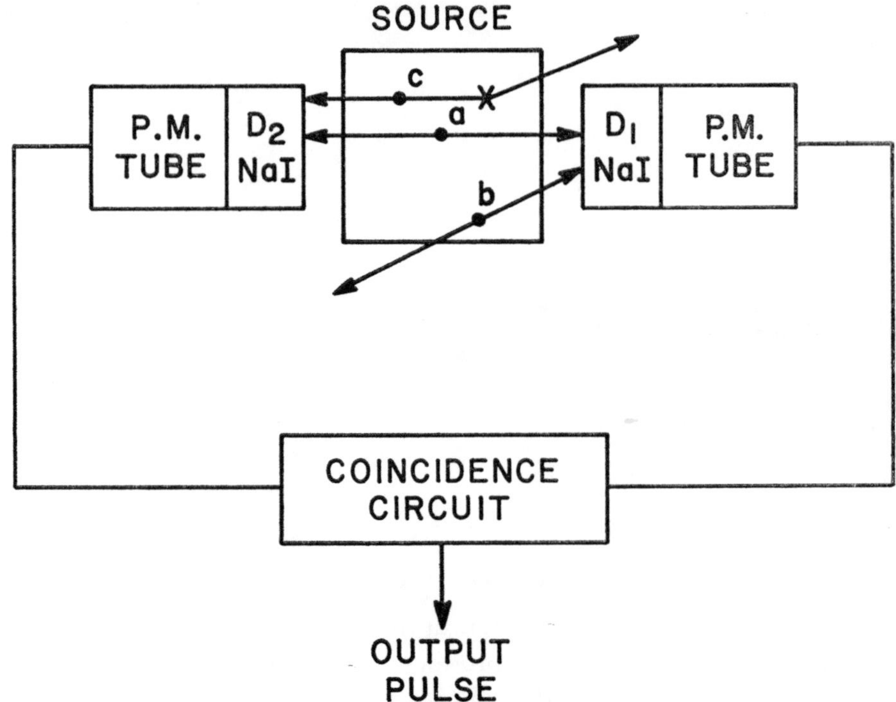


Figure 8-1. Coincidence detection of annihilation radiation. Event (a) is detected as a true coincidence. Events (b) and (c) may cause random coincidence.

and (c) will not result in a coincidence count individually. However, if the events (b) and (c) occur within the resolving time of the coincidence unit, they would be counted as a single coincidence count which is a chance or random count. The chance coincidence count rate should be much lower than the true coincidence count rate for statistically reliable imaging. The chance coincidence count rate is proportional to the coincidence resolving time and the singles count rate in each detector.

Positron cameras offer several advantages. It is possible to obtain good resolution without the use of collimators. Since the sum of the distances travelled by the two photons is the same, no matter where the annihilation event occurred, the spatial resolution is depth-independent. Therefore, lesions deep within the body can be detected as easily as those on the surface. The instruments that detect single gamma rays do not have this property. The background count rate is extremely low, which permits long exposures with little activity. Finally, positron cameras also have tomographic capability.

The disadvantage of this imaging device is that it is expensive due to the complex nature of the instrumentation. Also, there is a limit to the amount of radioactive material that can be administered to the patient since very high count rates can overload the detectors. Also, the availability of positron-emitting radionuclides is limited.

The maximum geometric resolution of the positron camera would be about 3 to 4 mm if the positron annihilates with an electron at the site of the nucleus emitting the positron. But the positron, emitted with some kinetic energy, travels a few millimeters before it comes to rest and annihilates with an electron. Hence, the annihilation photons are produced at the end of the positron path and therefore there is a loss of resolution. This loss in spatial resolution for 1 MeV positrons in soft tissue is about 2 to 3 mm. Thus the overall resolution of the positron camera is about 7 mm and is depth-independent.

The availability of on-site medical cyclotrons to produce unique short-lived positron-emitting radionuclides such as $^{11}$C (20 minutes), $^{13}$N (10 minutes) and $^{15}$O (2 minutes) will increase the usefulness of positron cameras in medical research.

Coincidence imaging of radionuclides emitting two photons in cascade is also possible with these detectors. However, unlike annihilation photons, cascade gamma rays are emitted isotopically, requiring a very long time to collect statistically enough counts in the image. Only a limited number of medically useful radionuclides emit photons in cascade.

## SEMICONDUCTOR DETECTORS

A detailed description of the mechanism of photon detection with semiconductor detectors is outside the scope of this book. Only the basic principle will be described here.

The electrons in atoms occupy discrete energy levels. When atoms are packed very closely, as in solids, the attractive forces of the other nuclei tend to smear out the discrete atomic energy levels, thus forming several discrete energy bands. The filling of the different energy bands by electrons determines the properties of the solids. In metals, the top energy band having electrons or the *valence band* is only partially filled. In semiconductors and insulators, the valence band is completely filled and the next allowed energy band or *conduction band* is completely empty, as shown in Figure 8-2, Part A. The energy bandgap between the conduction and the valence bands is large in insulators when compared to that of semiconductors. Thus, in semiconductors, electrons can be easily excited to the higher band.

When a photon enters a semiconductor, the energy of the photon is absorbed in the usual manner, i.e. by either photoelectric, Compton, or pair production interaction. The electrons produced by the primary inter-

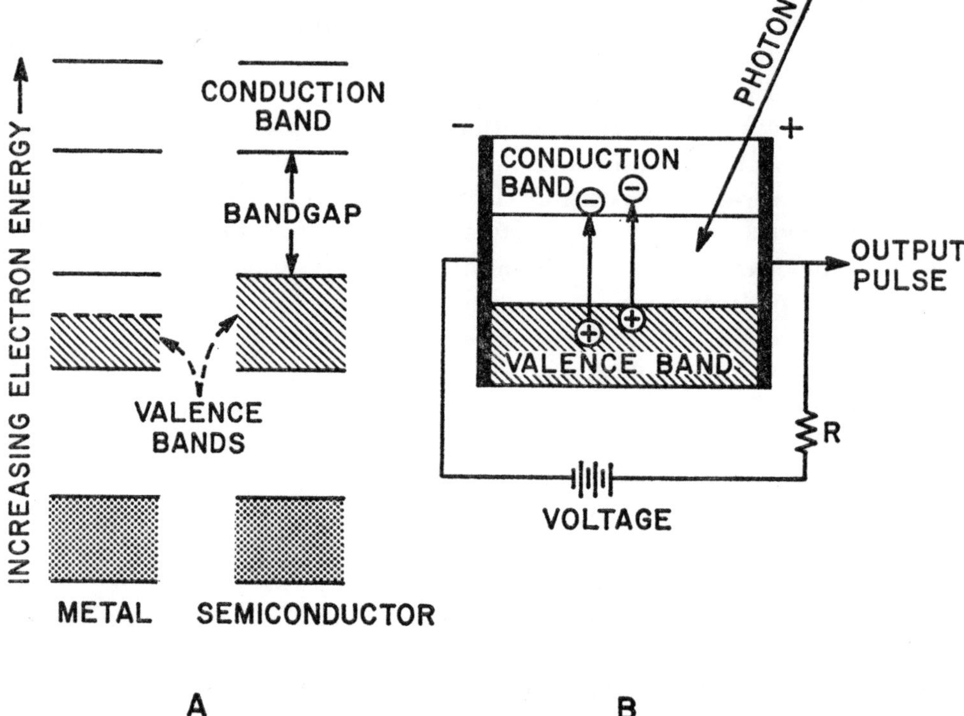


Figure 8-2. A.: Simplified energy-band structure for metals and semiconductors.
B.: Simple semiconductor model, illustrating the effect of radiation absorption.

action of photons with the semiconductor material transfer their energy to the valence electrons, thus elevating them into the conduction band. This leaves equal numbers of holes in the valence band, as shown in Fig. 8-2, Part B. These holes in the sea of electrons act as positively charged particles. If a voltage is applied across the semiconductor, the electrons in the conduction band move towards the positive electrode and the holes in the valence band move towards the negative electrode. Since the number of electron-hole pairs produced is proportional to the energy of the incident photon, the collection of the charges on the respective electrodes results in a pulse whose height is proportional to the photon energy. This pulse can be amplified and energy-discriminated for counting.

Germanium and silicon are well-known semiconductors. Important characteristics of these detectors are that they do not require photomultiplier tubes and their energy resolution is very good, approximately twenty times better than that of scintillation detectors. This is partly due to the small amount of energy needed by a germanium detector to form an electron-hole pair when compared to a scintillation detector. About 3 eV of energy is required to produce a pair in a germanium detector while 30 eV of energy is needed in a NaI detector. The excellent energy resolution offered by these semiconductor detectors improves the spatial resolution of the image, since many of the scattered photons can be eliminated by energy discrimination.

These detectors must be cooled to the temperature of liquid nitrogen for efficient operation. Another limitation of these detectors is that they are very expensive due to the difficulty of producing high-purity germanium crystal. Scanners and small position-sensitive detectors with germanium have been built and tested with promising results.

## GAS-FILLED DETECTORS

Radiation can be detected using a gas as the detection medium. A cathode wire and an anode wire are placed inside a chamber which is filled with a gas as shown in Figure 8-3. A voltage is applied across the electrode wires. Radiations entering the chamber will produce negative and positive ion pairs which are collected on the respective electrodes. The collection of charges on the electrodes can be used to detect the radiation.

IONIZATION CHAMBER. For low voltages, some of the ions produced by the radiations will recombine to form neutral atoms and some will be collected by the electrodes. As the voltage is increased, the free electrons will have less time to recombine with the positive ions since the electrons will be collected by the positive electrode more quickly and therefore the pulse height increases. At some voltage almost all ion pairs produced are collected. However, the pulse height is not enough to detect individual radiations, but the sum of all the events will result in a current which can be measured. The voltage range for which the output current is constant is called the *saturation region*. In this region, all the primary ions are collected without recombination. A gas detector with an applied voltage in the saturation region is called an *ionization chamber*. The variation of the pulse size with the applied voltage is also shown in Figure 8-3.

PROPORTIONAL COUNTER. If the applied voltage is increased beyond the saturation region, the ions moving towards the electrodes acquire enough energy to cause further ionization, thus increasing the pulse size. The pulse size is proportional to the energy of the radiation absorbed by the gas in this region. This voltage range is called the *proportional region*. The advantage of a proportional counter is that the pulses produced can be used to detect individual radiations and determine their energy.

GEIGER-MÜLLER COUNTER. Increasing the applied voltage still further increases the pulse size. In the Geiger-Müller region, the ionization occurs

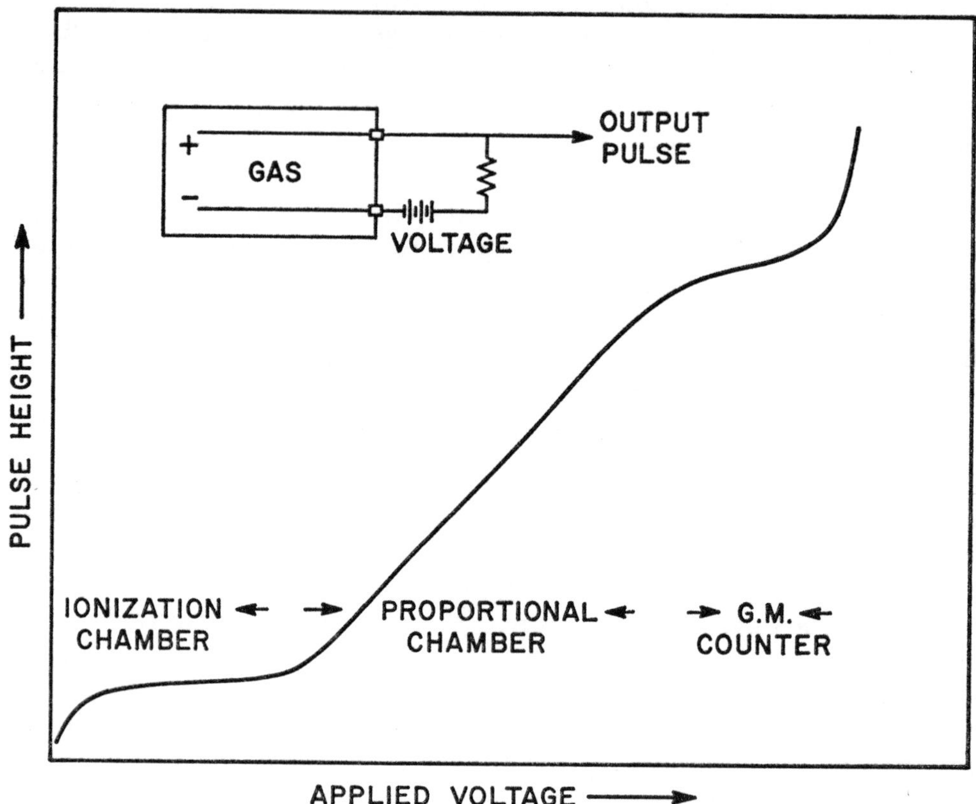


Figure 8-3. Pulse height as a function of applied voltage to a gas detector.

throughout the gas chamber and the ion amplification is of the order of a million or more. The output pulse size is independent of the energy of the ionizing event and therefore the pulses are of the same size for all different radiation. The voltage at which this process starts is called the *threshold voltage.* If the applied voltage is increased beyond the upper limit of the Geiger-Müller region, the detection of radiation is not possible due to continuous discharge in the gas. The Geiger-Müller counter, like the proportional counter, can be used to detect individual ionizing events, but cannot determine their energy.

## MULTIWIRE PROPORTIONAL CHAMBERS

Since proportional counters can discriminate the energy of the photons and can be used to count individual events, position-sensitive proportional chambers are being developed for nuclear medicine imaging. Scanners with a single wire and stationary imaging devices with large numbers of wires are being constructed and tested. In the stationary imaging device, the anode plane consists of an array of gold-plated tungsten wire with a spacing of 1.5 mm. The cathode planes are also made of tungsten wire with a spacing of 1 mm. The two cathode planes have their wires oriented at 90 degrees to each other and are on opposite sides of the anode. The cathode planes are operated at a negative voltage relative to the anode and therefore collect the positive ions. The chamber is filled with a 93 percent xenon and 7 percent $Co_2$ gas mixture.

The images obtained with a multiwire proportional chamber show excellent spatial resolution, about 1 mm in phantoms. Since the stopping power of the xenon gas is low at atmospheric pressure, the counting efficiency of the detector is also low. Increasing the pressure to 4 atmospheres increases the efficiency considerably. Besides the excellent spatial resolution, another advantage of this imaging device is that it can be inexpensive when compared to the conventional scintillation camera. It is also possible to construct a large whole-body stationary imaging detector.

The only disadvantage of the multiwire proportional counter is that its detection efficiency for 140 keV photons of [99m]Tc is low, even at a pressure of 4 atmospheres. Therefore, radionuclides emitting photons of energy less than 100 keV are needed for efficient imaging. The radionuclides emitting low-energy photons, such as [165]Er (50 keV), [177]Ta (55 keV), [195m]Pt (67 keV), [197]Hg (70 keV), and [201]Tl (70 keV), can be useful for efficient imaging although the tissue absorption will be more when compared to 140 keV photons. In fact the radionuclide [165]Er seems to be an ideal radionuclide to image with these detectors. Increasing the pressure of the xenon gas to 10 atmospheres might make [99m]Tc also a useful radionuclide with these promising detectors.

## TRANSMISSION AND FLUORESCENT IMAGING

TRANSMISSION IMAGING. The basic principle of transmission imaging is the same as in radiography. A radionuclide emitting monoenergetic photons is used in transmission imaging instead of an X-ray tube. Any of the previously mentioned detectors, i.e. NaI (Tl) detectors, Ge (Li) detectors or proportional counters can be used in principle to detect the transmitted photons. Scanners as well as stationary imaging devices can be utilized. Good collimation of the detector as well as the source is essential for good results.

A source and detector arrangement for transmission imaging is shown in Figure 8-4. Radionuclides for transmission imaging preferably should have long half-lives and emit photons of a single energy. The energy of the photon should be such that it gives enough penetration and good image

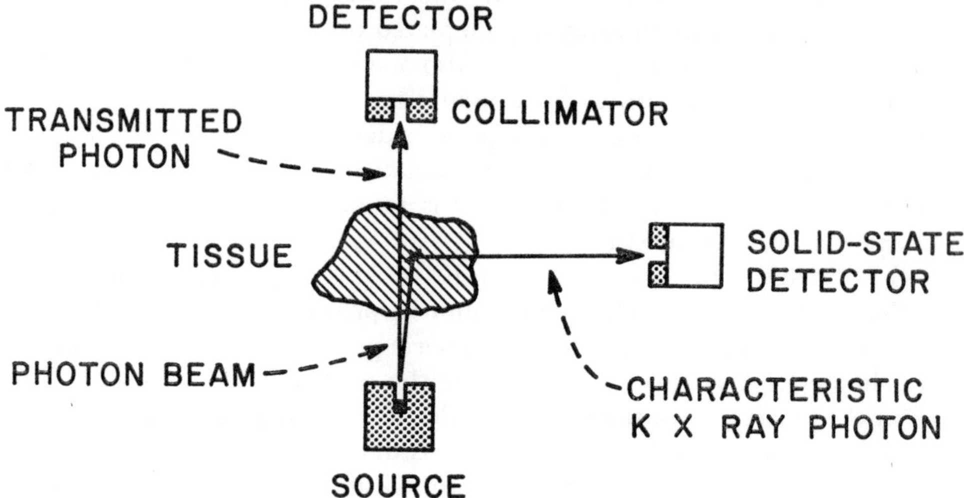


Figure 8-4. Principle of transmission and fluorescent imaging is illustrated. Solid-state detector shown at 90 degrees to the excitation beam is to detect the characteristic K x rays in fluorescent imaging.

contrast. The radionuclides generally used are $^{125}$I (28 keV), $^{241}$Am (60 keV) and $^{57}$Co (122 keV). For many organs, the radionuclide $^{159}$Dy (44 keV) may offer reasonably good contrast and sensitivity.

Transmission images are usually obtained to identify the patient anatomy in conjunction with emission images for diagnosis.

FLUORESCENT IMAGING. When a photon is absorbed by the photoelectric interaction, an electron from the K shell of the atom is ejected, leaving a vacancy in that shell. The transition of a higher orbital electron to the K shell usually results in the emission of characteristic K x rays, called *fluorescent radiation*. However, the photon energy should be higher than the binding energy of the K electron. The K x rays, thus emitted, can be used for imaging the distribution of an element in the organ of interest. For example, the thyroid image, i.e. the distribution of iodine in the thyroid, can be obtained by imaging with iodine K x rays (28 keV). The excitation of iodine atoms is achieved by using an external beam of photons from a monoenergetic source whose energy is higher than 28 keV.

A source and detector arrangement for fluorescent imaging is shown in Figure 8-4. The detector is placed at 90 degrees or more to the direction of the photon beam to avoid the interference from the transmitted photons. In order to eliminate the photons scattered into the detector from the original beam, a high-resolution detector such as a silicon detector must be used. The 60 keV photons from a $^{241}$Am source can be used to excite

K-shell fluorescence in the tissue elements whose K-electron binding energy is less than 60 keV.

The advantage of the transmission and the fluorescent imaging techniques is that the radiation dose to the patient is very low since the administration of radiopharmaceuticals to the patient is not involved in these procedures. The disadvantage of fluorescent imaging techniques is that only elements with high atomic number can be used for this purpose, and the only element with high enough concentration is iodine in thyroid tissue.

## ADDITIONAL READING

### Positron Camera

Hine, G.J.: Instrumentation in Nuclear Medicine. New York, Acad Pr, 1967, Vol. I.

### Solid State Detectors

Hoffer, P.B., Beck, R.N., Gottschalk, A.: Semiconductor Detectors in the Future of Nuclear Medicine. New York, Society of Nuclear Medicine, Inc., 1971.

### Multiwire Proportional Chamber

Kaufman, L., Perez-Mendez, V., Stoker, G.: Performance of a pressurized xenon-filled multiwire proportional chamber, IEEE *Trans Nucl Sci,* 20:426, 1973.
Borkowski, C.J., Kopp, M.K.: Proportional counter photon camera, IEEE *Trans Nucl Sci, 19:*161, 1972.
Borkowski, C.J., Kopp, M.K., Harter, J.A.: Line scanning proportional counter camera. IEEE *Trans Nucl Sci, NS-22:*896, 1975.
Rao, D.V., Goodwin, P.N., Khalil, F.L.: [165]Er: an ideal radionuclide for imaging with multiwire proportional gamma camera, *J. Nucl Med, 15:*1008, 1974.

### Transmission and Fluorescent Imaging

Hine, G.J., Sorenson, J.A.: Instrumentation in Nuclear Medicine. New York, Acad Pr, 1974, Vol. II.
Hoffer, P.B., Beck, R.N., Gottschalk, A.: *Semiconductor Detectors in the Future of Nuclear Medicine.* New York, Society of Nuclear Medicine, Inc., 1971.

## QUESTIONS

1. The positron camera detects
   (A) positrons of the same energy in coincidence.
   (B) a positron in coincidence with a photon.
   (C) photons of different energy in coincidence.
   (D) annihilation photons in coincidence.
2. The main advantage of the positron camera is that
   (A) it is simple to construct.
   (B) it gives depth-independent resolution.

(C)  it is inexpensive.
(D)  it can use many radionuclides for imaging.

3. In solid-state detectors, the interaction of photons results in the production of
    (A)  positive and negative ions.
    (B)  electron-hole pairs.
    (C)  scintillations.
    (D)  electron avalanches.

4. The main advantage of a germanium detector is that
    (A)  it is inexpensive.
    (B)  it is possible to develop a large whole-body camera.
    (C)  the detection efficiency for medium-energy photons is high.
    (D)  it offers better energy resolution.

5. Proportional counters are capable of detecting
    (A)  individual photons and their energy.
    (B)  only alpha and beta rays.
    (C)  individual photons but not their energy.
    (D)  only the dose rate.

6. In the Geiger-Müller counters, the pulse height is high enough to
    (A)  determine the energy of the event.
    (B)  count individual radiations.
    (C)  count and determine the energy of the radiations.
    (D)  cause continuous discharge.

7. The disadvantage of the multiwire proportional chamber for imaging is that
    (A)  the detection efficiency is low for 140 keV photons.
    (B)  it is too expensive.
    (C)  it offers poor spatial resolution.
    (D)  only small-size detectors are possible.

8. The ideal energy for imaging with xenon gas-filled multiwire proportional chambers is about
    (A)  511 keV.
    (B)  140 keV.
    (C)  50 keV.
    (D)  27 keV.

9. Fluorescent imaging of the thyroid can be done by detecting
    (A)  transmitted photons.
    (B)  scattered photons.
    (C)  photons from the excitation source.
    (D)  K x rays of iodine.

# Radionuclides in nuclear medicine

There are now more than 1500 radionuclides, counting both those naturally occurring and those capable of being produced. Only a relatively very few of these are useful in nuclear medicine. What are these radionuclides, what are the properties that make them useful, and how may such nuclides be produced? These are the questions which will be discussed briefly in this chapter.

## PHYSICAL PROPERTIES

Physical properties include the type of decay and the radiations emitted, the energy of the radiations, and the half-life.

DECAY SCHEMES AND RADIATIONS. The choice of radionuclide depends to some extent on the type of detection being used. For external detection of internally administered radionuclides, fairly high-energy x or gamma rays are required. As discussed in Chapter 3, gamma rays are usually emitted following decay by alpha or beta emission or electron capture. As for alpha emitters, the alpha particle yields a high radiation dose if used internally, cannot be detected *in vivo,* and is difficult to accurately count *in vitro.* Furthermore, there is generally a low yield of gamma radiation. Thus alpha emitters can be automatically excluded from consideration.

Many radionuclides which decay by $\beta^-$ emission emit suitable gamma rays. Two examples are $^{131}$I and $^{203}$Hg. However, with a beta-gamma emitter, most of the radiation dose is contributed by the beta particles, which places a limit on the number of millicuries which can be routinely administered. The same applies to beta-positive decay, although some positron-emitting radionuclides, such as $^{15}$O and $^{13}$N have been used, and advantage made of the fact that all positron emitters also emit two annihilation photons, each 0.511 MeV, in opposite directions. Other positron emitters, such as $^{18}$F, have been used since their short half-life limits the radiation dose received by the patient.

With some radionuclides which decay by beta-gamma emission, the product nuclides remain in the excited state a finite time before emitting a gamma photon and dropping to the ground state. If the product nuclide can be physically separated from its parent while in the excited or "metastable" state, then it is possible to obtain an almost pure gamma emitter; the chief example is technetium-99m. This and other parent-daughter relations will be further discussed in the last section of this chapter.

Another source of almost pure gamma emitters is those radionuclides which decay by electron capture, since this process is generally followed by gamma emission, as discussed in Chapter 3. Some examples are $^{75}$Se, $^{125}$I, and $^{197}$Hg.

In summary, the most desirable radionuclides from the standpoint of the decay scheme are those which decay by IT, isomeric transition (such as $^{99m}$Tc) , and EC, electron capture.

GAMMA ENERGY. Radionuclides are available having gamma rays with energies from a few keV up to several MeV; however, only part of this range is useful. Below about 25 keV, absorption in tissue becomes too great for good external detection; for example, at 30 keV, 50 percent of the photons are absorbed by only 2 cm of soft tissue, while at 20 keV the half-value thickness is less than 1 cm. Also, when using a gamma camera as the detector, photons of 50 keV or more are needed in order to produce enough light photons for good positional information. Actually, the resolution begins to deteriorate below about 75 keV, but imaging of sources down to about 50 keV is still possible.

At the upper end of the range, the efficiency of detection begins to drop, even for large sodium iodine crystals, as was shown in Figure 5-9. Also, problems of shielding and collimator construction increase rapidly, so that 500 or 600 keV is considered a practical upper limit. For gamma cameras, the maximum intrinsic resolution occurs in the region of 200 to 400 keV, but here the sensitivity is less because of the decrease in counting efficiency, as was shown in Figure 7-3, and because of the increased amount of lead needed for collimation. Thus the maximum sensitivity, while still maintaining good resolution, is only obtained in the region below about 150 keV.

It is also desirable that a gamma-emitting radionuclide emit photons of only one energy. Otherwise it may be difficult to exclude scattered radiation by pulse height analysis, since scattered photons from high-energy gamma rays may appear in the window which is being used to count low or medium-energy photons. Despite this, several nuclides which emit multiple gamma rays, such as $^{75}$Se and $^{67}$Ga have been used, but chiefly because of their desirable physiological properties, i.e. their action as tracers.

In summary, gamma emitters are most useful in the range from 25 to 600 keV, while for gamma camera use, the ideal range is only from about 75 to 150 keV.

HALF-LIFE. The list of available nuclides includes those with half-lives ranging from fractions of a second to thousands of years. Which half-lives are desirable or acceptable depends on the use being made of the radio-nuclides. For *in vitro* work, half-lives of days are usually needed, while half-lives of several weeks or a few months may be desirable in order to complete lengthy studies, or as a convenience in having the radionuclide available for repeated studies. However, the longer the half-life, the greater the problems of disposal and possible contamination of laboratories and equipment. Despite this, a few very long-lived radionuclides are widely used (for example, $^{14}$C, half-life 5730 years), but only because no other suitable isotopes of those elements are readily available.

For internal administration, short half-life radionuclides are desirable, since the shorter the half-life, the less the radiation dose per millicurie. Thus if the radiation dose to the patient is a limiting factor, the shorter half-lives allow more millicuries to be administered, resulting in higher counting rates. However, this argument can only be carried so far; if the half-life is too short, then most of the radionuclides may have decayed before it is taken up by the organ or tissue to be imaged. The ideal half-life for maximum counts with minimum total dose depends to some extent on the rate of uptake and the distribution and rate of elimination of that fraction which is not taken up; but in general, the most desirable half-life is one which lies between one and two times the time required for adequate uptake. For example, if a brain-scanning agent reaches a suitable concentration in three hours, then the half-life for such a radionuclide should be between three and six hours.

In summary, desirable half-lives are:

*In vitro:* a few days to a few months.

*In vivo:* a few hours to a few days.

## BIOLOGICAL PROPERTIES

The selection of a radionuclide also involves the question of the biological behavior of the element or the compound of which the element is a part. There are three ways in which radionuclides may be used in nuclear medicine: (1) selecting an element which has the desired biological properties, such as a propensity to concentrate in an organ or structure, and using one of the radioisotopes of that element, (2) selecting a compound having the desirable properties, and synthesizing that compound using a radioisotope of an element normally present in the compound, or (3) taking a compound which has the desired biological behavior, and tagging it with a radionuclide which has the desirable physical properties, i.e. those properties discussed in the previous section.

The principle example of the first type is iodine, which concentrates so strongly in the thyroid. There are more than twenty radioisotopes of iodine available, of which six or eight have reasonable half-lives. The most widely used isotope of iodine has been $^{131}$I, but only because of its availability and low cost; as a beta-gamma emitter with an eight-day half-life, it is not desirable from a physical standpoint. A more ideal choice would be $^{123}$I, with a twelve-hour half-life and a 159 keV gamma ray. Should $^{123}$I become more widely available, it may largely replace $^{131}$I in clinical use.

Examples of the second type are the various agents used for renal studies, such as chlormerodrin, which was first synthesized using $^{203}$Hg in place of the stable mercury atom. Subsequently, $^{197}$Hg has been used because of its shorter half-life and decay by electron capture. Other examples include the production of human serum albumin using $^{131}$I, and the synthesis of methionine using $^{75}$Se in place of a sulfur atom, yielding selenomethionine, useful for pancreatic scanning.

The most widely used example of the third type of radiopharmaceutical is $^{99m}$Tc, which in the pertechnetate form can be readily tagged to other compounds, such as sulfur colloids or serum albumin. Its physical properties are so ideal that new attempts are continually being made to tag additional compounds with it; for example, a large number of bone-localizing agents are now available, tagged with $^{99m}$Tc. The production of $^{99m}$Tc will be discussed in a later section, but the properties of $^{99m}$Tc are such that it is tending to largely replace most other radionuclides, at least for *in vivo* imaging.

## THE PRODUCTION OF RADIONUCLIDES

There are four principal sources or methods for obtaining radioactive nuclides for nuclear medicine. These are (1) fission products from a nuclear reactor, (2) neutron activation in a nuclear reactor, (3) cyclotron production, and (4) parent-daughter generators. Some of the commonly used radionuclides may be produced by any of several different methods or reactions. Each of the four principal methods will now be described and some possible examples given.

FISSION PRODUCTS. The process of nuclear fission may be briefly described as follows: If a relatively rare isotope of uranium, $^{235}$U, captures a neutron, the resulting nucleus, $^{236}$U, is highly unstable; but instead of losing energy by alpha or beta decay, it splits into two nuclei of approximately equal mass, plus two or three high-speed neutrons. In a typical nuclear reactor, enriched uranium, that is, uranium containing more than the usual percentage of $^{235}$U, is used together with some moderating substance, a light element such as graphite or "heavy" water (water containing $^{2}$H) which serves to slow down the neutrons so they may be more easily captured by other $^{235}$U nuclei. Also present is some neutron-absorbing substance, such as cadmium rods; the amount present may be adjusted to keep the chain reaction going at the desired power level. Plutonium 239, which undergoes fission after capture of a slow neutron, is also widely used as a fuel for nuclear reactors.

The two medium-weight elements resulting from nuclear fission are known as *fission products*. The $^{235}$U nucleus does not split exactly in two, but produces two elements whose masses have a ratio of about 0.6. Figure 9-1 shows the relative amounts of the various elements produced in the fission of $^{235}$U.

The stable isotopes of medium and heavy elements have more neutrons than protons, and the heavier the element, the larger the neutron-proton ratio. Thus if a very heavy element like uranium undergoes fission, the resulting products will be neutron-rich, i.e. have too many neutrons for stability. As discussed in Chapter 3, a nucleus may reduce its neutron-proton ratio by negative beta decay. Thus the fission products are almost

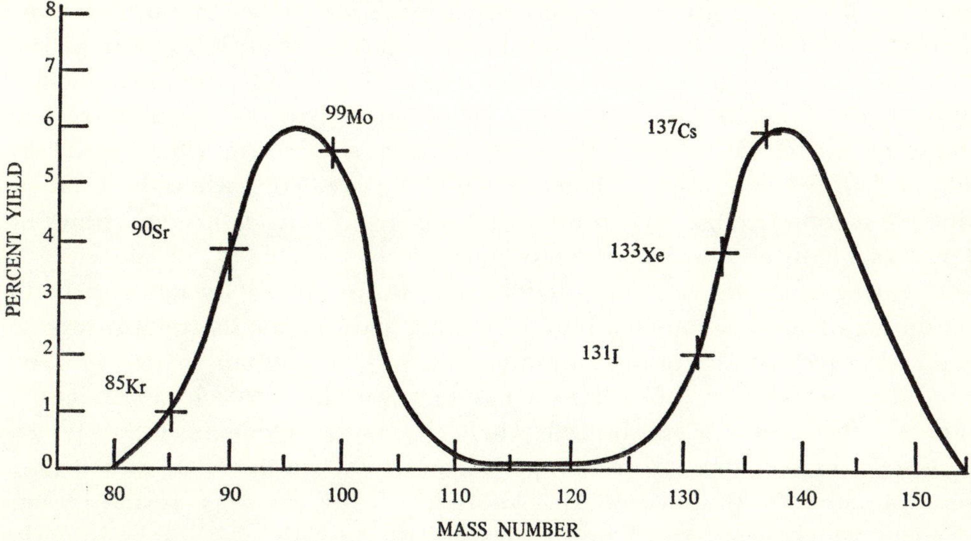


Figure 9-1. The relative amounts of some of the fission products resulting from the fission of $^{235}$U.

all beta emitters, or beta-gamma emitters, often requiring several successive beta decays to reach stability.

After a certain time in the reactor, some of the uranium or plutonium fuel may be removed and any desirable fission products separated out by chemical means. This was an early source of $^{131}I$ for medical use, and a source of $^{90}Sr$ and $^{137}Cs$, among others. Recently, $^{99}Mo$ has also been obtained in this manner. Although many radioactive elements are produced as fission products, chemical separation is often complicated by the presence of other isotopes of the desired element, and other methods of production are sometimes preferred.

NEUTRON BOMBARDMENT. As mentioned above, the fission process releases fast neutrons which are subsequently slowed down. Almost any nucleus has the ability to capture a low-energy or *thermal* neutron; in general, the lower the neutron energy, the greater the probability of capture, although some elements have resonances at a particular neutron energy where the probability of capture is unusually high. The probability that a nucleus will capture a bombarding neutron is known as the capture *cross section,* and has the dimensions of an area which may be thought of as representing the apparent size of the target seen by a bombarding neutron. Thus a large value for the cross section means that there is a high probability of capturing a neutron.

A nuclear reactor intended for radioisotope production contains several access ports, or hollow tubes leading into the core of the reactor so that suitably prepared target elements may be placed in a region of high neutron flux. The time required for irradiation depends on the cross section, the neutron flux, and the desired specific activity, as well as the half-life of the resulting radionuclide. The activity of the product nuclide approaches a maximum value after six or seven half-lives because of the decay of nuclei already produced. Typically, irradiation times equal to several half-lives are used, although for high-flux reactors, when the product nuclide is long-lived, or when only low specific activity is needed, times of less than a half-life may be more economical.

A large number of radionuclides may be produced by neutron bombardment of stable elements. However, since most elements contain several stable isotopes, undesirable radionuclides, or contaminants, may also be produced, which are difficult to separate from the desired radionuclide. These difficulties are minimized when the target element has only, or consists of mostly, one stable isotope; for example, stable $^{197}Au$, which may be irradiated to produce $^{198}Au$. Another convenient way is to use an element which when irradiated forms a radionuclide which subsequently decays into the desired radionuclide. For example, stable $^{130}Te$ may be irradiated, forming $^{131}Te$, which decays by beta emission to $^{131}I$, which may then be chemically separated from the Te. This is the method which has been most commonly used for producing [131]I for medical use. Other reactor-produced radionuclides include [24]Na, [32]P, [60]Co, [75]Se, [125]I, and [197]Hg. Since neutron bombardment adds a neutron to the nucleus, most reactor-produced radionuclides decay by $\beta^-$ emission, although a few, such as [197]Hg, decay by electron capture.

CYCLOTRON PRODUCTION. Nuclear reactors have long been an abundant and inexpensive source of many radionuclides; however, as discussed in the first part of this chapter, radionuclides which decay by beta or beta-gamma emissions are less desirable for internal administration than those which decay by electron capture or isomeric transition; also, since almost all fission products and most reactor-produced radionuclides decay by beta or beta-gamma, some other methods of radionuclide production are desirable. In order for a nucleus to decay by positron emission, or by electron capture, which is often an alternative to $\beta^+$ decay, one or more protons must be added to the nucleus. Furthermore, protons having energies of many MeV must be used in order to overcome the repulsion between positively charged protons and the positively charged nucleus. This requires some form of charged-particle accelerator, of which there are a number of different types, such as cyclotrons, synchrocyclotrons, proton-synchrotrons, etc. However, most of the radionuclides produced for medical use have been obtained using relatively small cyclotrons, since the required energy of 5 to 30 MeV can be obtained with these machines. Also, since many of the cyclotron-produced products have very short half-lives, it is desirable to use a machine which can be located close to where the radionuclides will be used. In fact, small cyclotrons have been located in or adjacent to a number of hospitals, including Hammersmith in London, Mallinckroft in St. Louis, and hospitals in Boston, New York, and Chicago. Several commercial companies also operate small cyclotrons for the production of radionuclides for medical use.

Although some radionuclides can be produced by either neutron bombardment or by the use of a cyclotron, the latter method may be preferred in order to obtain carrier-free and/or high-specific-activity radionuclides.

The principle of operation of a cyclotron is a relatively simple one, first developed by E. O. Lawrence in 1932. Positively charged particles move in circular orbits of increasing size; a magnetic field, at right angles to the plane of the orbits, keeps the particles going in circular fashion, while electrostatic forces are used to accelerate the particles every time they cross gaps between segments of the circular chamber in which they are moving. The particles move in ever larger orbits until they come out of the machine as a beam and strike an external target. In addition to protons ([1]H), deuterons ([2]H), helium 3 ions ([3]He), and helium 4 ions ([4]He) are also used as beam sources in cyclotrons. A large number of elements have been used as targets; in many cases, the target nucleus loses one or more neutrons when hit by the positive particle. Thus the production of a wide variety of radionuclides is possible, depending on the choice of particle and the choice of target.

Among the medically useful radionuclides produced by cyclotron bombardment are $^{15}O$, produced by deutrons on $^{14}N$; and $^{18}F$, produced by $^3He$ ions or alpha particles on water ($^{16}O$). Other cyclotron-produced radionuclides include $^{57}Co$, $^{67}Ga$, $^{123}I$, and $^{127}Xe$.

PARENT-DAUGHTER GENERATORS. Short-lived radionuclides are desirable for most *in vivo* procedures, as discussed in the first part of this chapter. For greatest convenience, the source of a short-lived radionuclide should be located close to the place of utilization and capable of supplying the radionuclide whenever needed. Such a situation may exist when a relatively long-lived radionuclide decays to form another radionuclide which has a short half-life. Many such parent-daughter relationships exist, but the one which has been most useful in nuclear medicine is the $^{99}Mo$- $^{99m}Tc$ combination. A simplified decay scheme was shown in Figure 3-3. $^{99}Mo$, with a half-life of 2.8 days, is available as a fission product, or may be produced by neutron bombardment of $^{98}Mo$. Fission product $^{99}Mo$ has the advantage that it may be obtained almost carrier free, i.e. containing no stable isotopes of Mo, and thus will have a high specific activity.

Most commercially available Mo-Tc generator systems are based on the principle of column chromatography, in which the molybdenum is absorbed on a suitable ion-exchange material, such as alumina, to form molybdate ions. When saline solution is passed through the column, the technetium atoms which have been formed from the decay of the $^{99}Mo$ are washed off, or *eluded,* in the form of pertechnetate ions, $TcO_4$, leaving $^{99}Mo$ still attached to the column. The specific activity of the pertechnetate depends on the number of millicuries of $^{99}Mo$ and the amount of saline needed to remove the $^{99m}Tc$. With high specific-activity $^{99}Mo$, i.e., high mCi/mg, less saline is needed, yielding higher specific-activity $^{99m}Tc$, i.e., high mCi/ml.

When the half-life of a daughter radionuclide is shorter than that of the parent, a state of equilibrium is reached in which the activities of each are approximately equal and appear to decay with the half-life of the parent. Thus a 100 mCi source of $^{99}Mo$ contains approximately 100 mCi of $^{99m}Tc$; although the $^{99m}Tc$ is decaying faster, new $^{99m}Tc$ nuclei are constantly being formed by the decay of the $^{99}Mo$. After removal of all of the $^{99m}Tc$ by eluding the generator, the build-up of new $^{99m}Tc$ in the generator will be rapid, but since some of the newly formed Tc nuclei are always decaying, the amount of $^{99m}$Tc present will increase approximately as

$$N_2 = N_1 \left(1 - e^{-\lambda_2 t}\right), \tag{9.1}$$

where $N_2$ = activity of $^{99m}$Tc, $N_1$ = activity of Mo, and $\lambda_2$ = the decay constant of $^{99m}$Tc.

The build-up and decay of $^{99m}$Tc and $^{99}$Mo are shown in Figure 9-2. The $^{99m}$Tc will reach one-half its maximum activity in about six hours, and three-fourths of its maximum in about twelve hours. The time for a parent-daughter combination to reach maximum equilibrium is given in the relation:

$$t = \frac{1}{\lambda_2 - \lambda_1} \ln \left[\frac{\lambda_2}{\lambda_1}\right], \tag{9.2}$$

where $\lambda_1$ and $\lambda_2$ are the decay constants of the parent and daughter respectively. Using equation (2.7), the decay constants are

$$^{99m}Tc: \quad \lambda_2 = \frac{0.693}{6.03 \text{ hr}} = 0.1149 \text{ hr}^{-1},$$

$$^{99}Mo: \quad \lambda_1 = \frac{0.693}{66.7 \text{ hr}} = 0.0104 \text{ hr}^{-1}.$$

Thus equation (9.2) gives

$$t = \frac{1}{0.1045} \ln (11.05) = 23 \text{ hr.}$$

Thereafter, if all the $^{99}$Mo atoms decayed to $^{99m}$Tc, then the activity of the daughter would slightly exceed that of the parent, as shown by the dotted line in Figure 9-2. This may be explained intuitively by saying that at any given time, some of the daughter nuclei present were formed when there was more parent present, since the half-life of the parent is not negligible compared to that of the daughter. However, in the case of $^{99}$Mo, only about 86 percent of the $^{99}$Mo atoms decay to $^{99m}$Tc (see Figure 3-3), so that the amount of $^{99m}$Tc remains less than the amount of $^{99}$Mo.

In practice, Mo-Tc generators are generally eluted every twenty-four hours, although substantial amounts of $^{99m}$Tc can be obtained more often if needed, as shown in Figure 9-2. Although a longer half-life for the parent would be desirable, the 67-hour half-life of $^{99}$Mo enables shipments to be made on a weekly basis; and the ideal properties of $^{99m}$Tc have made Mo-Tc generators the most widely used source of radionuclides for nuclear medicine.

A large number of **parent-daughter generator combinations** are possible but only one other has been widely used in nuclear medicine, and that is the $^{113}$Sn-$^{113m}$In generator. The radionuclide $^{113}$Sn is produced by neutron bombardment of $^{112}$Sn, and absorbed on a zirconium-oxide ion-exchange

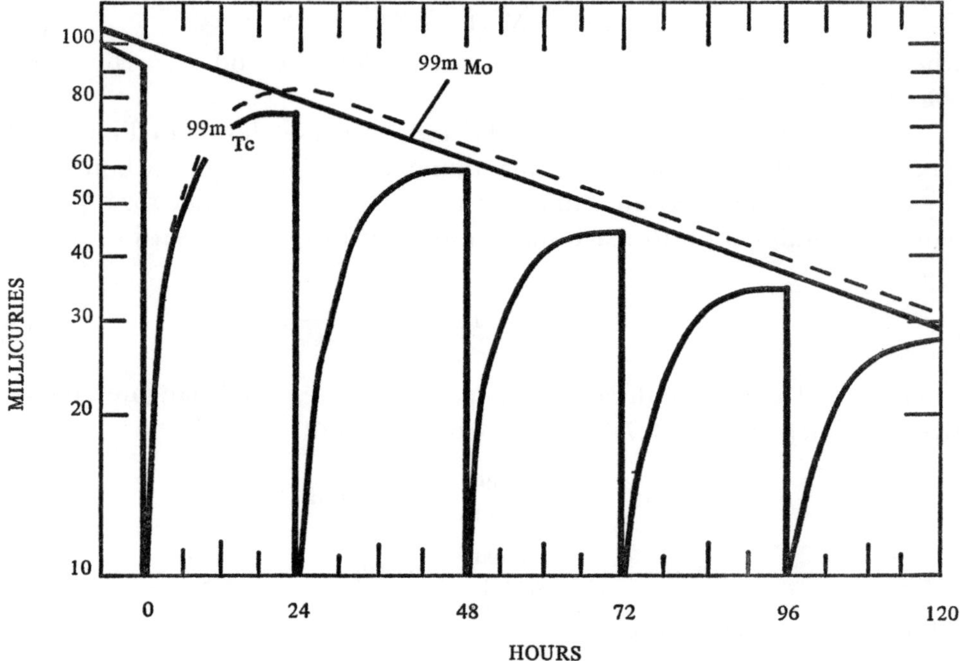


Figure 9-2. Plot of the build-up and decay of 99mTc in a generator which contains 100 mCi of 99Mo at the time of eluding. The dotted curve shows what the build-up would be if all the 99Mo decayed to 99mTc; actually about 14 percent bypass the isomeric state (see Figure 3-3).

column. The 113mIn may be eluded by a dilute acid and used in the ionic form, or converted to form colloids and chelates. The advantages include the long half-life of the parent (115 days), and the very short half-life of the daughter (100 minutes), which decays by isomeric transition, thus giving a low patient dose. Disadvantages include the fact that the 393 keV photon is less efficiently detected and collimated by gamma cameras than is the 140 keV photon from 99mTc.

Other generators which have been developed and used for nuclear medicine, at least on an experimental basis, include 81Rb-81mKr, with half-lives of 4.7 hours and 13 seconds, respectively, and 82Sr-82Rb, with half-lives of 25 days and 1.3 minutes, respectively. It is possible that with the completion of new isotope production facilities now being planned in connection with the new high-intensity-beam particle accelerators at Brookhaven and Los Alamos, these and other generator systems may become more widely available.

## QUESTIONS

1. The most desirable radionuclides for external detection are those which decay by
   (A) alpha emission.
   (B) beta-gamma emission.
   (C) positron emission.
   (D) electron capture and isomeric transitions.

2. The most desirable gamma energies for external detection by gamma cameras are
   (A) less than 50 keV.
   (B) 75-150 keV.
   (C) 200-400 keV.
   (D) greater than 500 keV.

3. For internal administration, the ideal half-life should be
   (A) as short as possible.
   (B) one or two times the uptake time.
   (C) several days.
   (D) a few days to a few months.

4. The fission of a uranium atom results in the formation of
   (A) radioisotopes of all elements.
   (B) mostly medium-atomic number radionuclides.
   (C) alpha particles only.
   (D) two stable elements.

5. Most fission-product nuclei decay by
   (A) alpha emission.
   (B) beta and beta-gamma emission.
   (C) positron emission.
   (D) electron capture.

6. Radionuclides produced by neutron bombardment in a nuclear reactor generally decay by
   (A) alpha emission.
   (B) positron emission.
   (C) electron capture and internal conversion.
   (D) beta and beta-gamma emission.

7. Cyclotron-produced radionuclides may be desirable because
   (A) they are cheaper.
   (B) they are always available.
   (C) they have longer half-lives.
   (D) they generally decay by electron capture.

8. In a parent-daughter generator, the amount of activity of the daughter present at equilibrium
   (A) depends on the half-life of the daughter.
   (B) remains constant.
   (C) continually increases exponentially.
   (D) is approximately equal to the activity of the parent.

# 10

# Statistics of radiation measurements

Experimental results are always to some extent variable. If an experiment is repeated, a somewhat different result may be obtained. Therefore no special importance can be attached to any single measurement. The science of statistics is useful to know the degree of accuracy of any single experiment. Statistics are the data that characterize a sample, and the half-life of a sample of radioactive atoms is an example of statistics. In this chapter only the statistics of radiation measurements are considered.

## STANDARD DEVIATION

Due to the random nature of radioactive decay, one cannot tell when a given atom will decay. The decay of atoms is independent of each other. Such processes are described by the *Poisson distribution*. The *standard deviation* for such a distribution is given by

$$\sigma = \sqrt{N} \qquad (10.1)$$

where $N$ is the number of events detected. If $N$ is the true mean, then the probability that a single count will lie between $N - \sqrt{N}$ and $N + \sqrt{N}$ is 67 percent and the probability that a single measurement will lie between $N - 2\sqrt{N}$ and $N + 2\sqrt{N}$ is 96 percent.

*Example 10.1:* In an experiment, 10,000 counts were obtained in a minute. Calculate the standard deviation and find 67 and 96 percent intervals for true mean value.

$$\text{standard deviation} = \sqrt{10,000} = 100$$
$$67\% \text{ interval} = 10,000 - 100 \text{ to } 10,000 + 100$$
$$= 9,900 \text{ to } 10,100.$$

This means if the experiment is repeated a hundred times, the chances are that sixty-seven of the measurements will be within the range of 9,900 to 10,100 and thirty-three will be outside the range.

$$96\% \text{ interval} = 10{,}000 - (2 \times 100) \text{ to } 10{,}000 + (2 \times 100)$$
$$= 9{,}800 \text{ to } 10{,}200$$

This means, out of a hundred measurements, ninety-six will be within the above range and four outside the range.

The *probable error P* is defined as

$$P = 0.67\, \sigma = 0.67\, \sqrt{N} \tag{10.2}$$

The probability that the true mean lies within $N \pm P$ is 50 percent.

*Example 10.2:* Calculate the probable error for 10,000 counts. The standard deviation as in example 10.1 is 100.

$$P = 0.67 \times 100 = 67$$

This means that if the experiment is repeated, the chances are 50 percent for the result to be within the range of 9,933 to 10,067.

The standard deviation, when expressed as the percentage of the total number of counts, is sometimes called *standard error (s.e.)* or *coefficient of variation.*

$$s.e. = \frac{\sigma}{N}\,100 = \frac{\sqrt{N}}{N}\,100 = \frac{100}{\sqrt{N}} \tag{10.3}$$

This decreases with increasing number of accumulated counts.

*Example 10.3:* Calculate the percent standard deviation for 1,000 and 10,000 counts.

$$\sigma \text{ for } 1{,}000 \text{ counts} = \sqrt{1{,}000} = 32$$
$$\% \text{ standard deviation} = \frac{100}{\sigma} = \frac{100}{32} = 3\%$$
$$\sigma \text{ for } 10{,}000 \text{ counts} = 100$$
$$\% \text{ standard deviation} = \frac{100}{100} = 1\%$$

*Example 10.4:* Find the number of counts required to obtain a standard error of 0.5 percent. From equation (10.3),

$$0.5 = \frac{100}{\sqrt{N}}$$

$$\sqrt{N} = \frac{100}{0.5} = 200$$

$$N = (200)^2 = 40{,}000 \text{ counts.}$$

The statistical uncertainty is less when the total number of counts is large as seen in the above examples. The number of counts required to achieve various degrees of accuracy is given in Table 10-I. High degrees of accuracy can be achieved with large numbers of counts. This may require either high activities or long counting times.

TABLE 10-I

STANDARD ERROR FOR DIFFERENT TOTAL NUMBERS OF COLLECTED COUNTS

| *Total No. of Counts* | *Standard Deviation* | *Standard Error (%)* |
|---|---|---|
| 100 | 10 | 10 |
| 500 | 22 | 4.5 |
| 1,000 | 32 | 3.1 |
| 2,000 | 45 | 2.2 |
| 4,000 | 63 | 1.6 |
| 10,000 | 100 | 1 |
| 20,000 | 141 | 0.7 |
| 40,000 | 200 | 0.5 |
| 100,000 | 316 | 0.3 |
| 400,000 | 632 | 0.16 |
| 1,000,000 | 1,000 | 0.1 |

This discussion so far is true only when the counting time is much shorter than the half-life of the radionuclide in question. This condition is usually satisfied for the radionuclides used in nuclear medicine, since the half-lives are much longer than the counting times for a procedure.

## BACKGROUND

The total counts obtained in an experiment are usually the sum of the counts due to the radiations originating from the sample of radioactivity and the counts arising from all other sources. These other sources are cosmic radiation coming from outer space, natural radioactivity from the materials in the walls and the radiations from other radioactive materials stored in the same or adjacent rooms. This background count can be obtained by removing the radioactive sample from the detector. The net count from the sample is then equal to the number of counts obtained with the radioactive sample minus the counts without the sample counted for the same time. If $N_s$ is the number of counts obtained with the sample and $N_b$ is the number of background counts for the same time, then the net count is

$$N_n = N_s - N_b. \qquad (10.4)$$

The standard deviation of the net count $N_n$ is not $\sqrt{N_n}$ as one might think. The standard deviation of $N_s$ and $N_b$ can be calculated in the usual way, i.e.

$$\sigma_s = \sqrt{N_s}$$
$$\sigma_b = \sqrt{N_b}.$$

Then, the standard deviation of the net count $N$ is given by

$$\sigma_n = \sqrt{\sigma_s^2 + \sigma_b^2}$$

$$\sigma_n = \sqrt{N_s + N_b}. \tag{10.5}$$

The standard error can be calculated using the formula

$$\% \text{ Standard error} = \frac{100\sigma_n}{N_n}. \tag{10.6}$$

*Example 10.5:* The background count is 100. The number of counts obtained in the same time with a sample of radioactivity is 1,000. Calculate the net count and standard deviation.

$$\text{Net count } N_n = N_s - N_b$$
$$= 1,000 - 100$$
$$= 900$$
$$\sigma_s = \sqrt{1,000} = 32$$
$$\sigma_b = \sqrt{100} = 10$$
$$\text{Standard deviation in } N_n = \sqrt{1,000 + 100}$$
$$= \sqrt{1,100}$$
$$= 33.$$

This is different from $\sqrt{N_n} = \sqrt{900} = 30$

*Example 10.6:* Calculate the standard error for the data given in example 10.5:

$$s.e. = \frac{100\sigma_n}{N_n}$$

$$= \frac{100 \times 33}{900}$$

$$= 3.7\%$$

If there is no background radiation at all, the sample count $N_s$ will be 900 counts. Then the $\%$ s.e. is

$$\frac{100}{\sqrt{N_n}} = \frac{100}{30} = 3.3.$$

Hence, the presence of the background radiation increases the statistical error.

It is sometimes convenient to analyze experimental data in terms of count rates. If $N_s$ and $N_b$ are the numbers of counts obtained with and without the sample respectively in a time $t_s$ and $t_b$, then the count rates $R_s$ and $R_b$ are

$$R_s = \frac{N_s}{t_s}; R_b = \frac{N_b}{t_b}. \tag{10.7}$$

Then, the net count rate $R_n$ is

$$R_n = R_s - R_b. \tag{10.8}$$

The standard deviation of a count rate is given by

$$\sigma_R = \sqrt{R/t}. \tag{10.9}$$

The standard deviation in the net count is then given by the equation

$$\sigma_n = \sqrt{\frac{R_s}{t_s} + \frac{R_b}{t_b}}. \tag{10.10}$$

The percent standard error can be calculated from

$$s.e. = \frac{100\sigma_n}{R_n}. \tag{10.11}$$

*Example 10.7:* When a sample of radioactivity was counted for 10 minutes, 2,000 counts were obtained. The background count gave 500 counts to five minutes. Calculate the (a) sample count rate, (b) background count rate, (c) net count rate, (d) standard deviation in the net count rate, (e) percent standard error.

(a) From equation (10.7)

$$R_s = \frac{N_s}{t_s}$$
$$= \frac{2000}{10}$$
$$= 200 \; cpm.$$

(b) From equation (10.7)

$$R_b = \frac{500}{5}$$
$$= 100 \; cpm.$$

(c) From equation (10.8)

$$R_n = 200 - 100$$
$$= 100 \; cpm.$$

(d) From equation (10.10)

$$\sigma_n = \sqrt{\frac{R_s}{t_s} + \frac{R_b}{t_b}}$$
$$= \sqrt{\frac{200}{10} + \frac{100}{5}}$$
$$= \sqrt{20 + 20}$$
$$= \sqrt{40}$$
$$= 6.3.$$

(e) From equation (10.11)

$$s.e. = \frac{100\sigma_n}{R_n}$$
$$= \frac{100 \times 6.3}{100}$$
$$= 6.3\%.$$

When the background count is much smaller than the sample count, then the net count is approximately equal to the sample count. Then the standard deviation for the net count rate can be obtained from equation (10.10) by taking $R_b \approx O$.

$$\sigma_n = \sqrt{\frac{R_s}{t_s}}; \; R_b \ll R_s. \tag{10.12}$$

The statistical accuracy increases with the increasing counting time when the background count rate is comparable to the sample count rate. This can be better explained with an example.

*Example 10.8:* In the previous example, if the counting time is increased by a factor of three, the sample counts and background counts will be 6000/30 minutes and 1500/15 minutes. The count rates are the same as in the previous example. Calculate the standard error.

$$s.e. = \frac{100\sigma_n}{R_n},$$

but

$$\sigma_n = \sqrt{\frac{R_s}{t_s} + \frac{R_b}{t_b}}.$$

Substituting for $\sigma_n$ gives

$$s.e. = \frac{100}{R_n} \sqrt{\frac{R_s}{t_s} + \frac{R_b}{t_b}}.$$
$$R_s = 200, \; t_s = 30 \text{ minutes}$$
$$R_b = 100, \; t_b = 15 \text{ minutes}$$
$$R_n = 200 - 100 = 100.$$
$$s.e. = \frac{100}{100} \sqrt{\frac{200}{30} + \frac{100}{15}}$$
$$= \sqrt{6.66 + 6.66}$$
$$= \sqrt{13.32}$$
$$= 3.6\%$$

The standard error calculated in the previous example (example 10.7) was 6.3 percent. Thus an increase in the counting time decreases the error.

When the background count rate is comparable to the sample count rate, long counting times are necessary to obtain the required degree of accuracy. The counting time for sample and background count will be minimum when they satisfy the following condition:

$$\frac{t_s}{t_b} = \sqrt{\frac{R_s}{R_b}} \qquad (10.13)$$

An example will illustrate this idea.

*Example 10.9:* What is the total minimum time required to obtain a standard error of 1 percent for the count rates given in example 10.7?

From example 10.7,

$$R_s = 200 \; cpm, \; R_b = 100 \; cpm, \; R_n = 100 \; cpm.$$

From equation (10.13),

$$\frac{t_s}{t_b} = \sqrt{\frac{200}{100}} = \sqrt{2} = 1.4$$

$$t_s = 1.4 \, t_b.$$

From equations (10.10) and (10.11),

$$s.e. = \frac{100}{R_n} \sqrt{\frac{R_s}{t_s} + \frac{R_b}{t_b}}.$$

Requiring s.e. to be 1 percent,

$$1 = \frac{100}{100} \sqrt{\frac{200}{1.4 t_b} + \frac{100}{t_b}}.$$

$$1 = \sqrt{\frac{200 + 140}{1.4 \, t_b}}.$$

Squaring both sides,

$$1 = \frac{340}{1.4 t_b}$$

$$t_b = \frac{340}{1.4} = 243 \text{ minutes;}$$

$$t_s = 1.4 \, t_b = 243 \times 1.4 = 340 \text{ minutes.}$$

The minimum total time required to obtain a standard error of 1 percent is $243 + 340 = 583$ minutes.

## RESOLVING TIME

All detectors require some time to detect an ionizing event. If another radiation enters the detector before the previous event is completely processed, that radiation will not be detected. Thus, the *resolving time* ($\tau$) or *dead time* is the time required between successive pulses if they are to be recorded separately. In other words, pulses closer than the resolving time are counted as one pulse resulting in a lost count. When the count rate becomes very high, the number of counts lost due to the dead time increases.

The resolving time of scintillation detectors is very small and usually of the order of a microsecond. For example, a detector may have a resolving time of 1 $\mu$sec. This detector can detect $10^6$ counts of radiation per second without loss of counts if all the radiations emitted are equally spaced in time. However, due to the random nature of the radioactive decay, the time interval between the events will not be the same for all radiations.

The resolving time $\tau$ can be determined experimentally by using two sources of approximately the same activity. If the number of counts per second is $R_A$ with source $A$, $R_B$ with source $B$, and $R_{AB}$ with sources $A$ and $B$ together, then the resolving time can be calculated from the equation

$$\tau = \frac{R_A + R_B - R_{AB}}{2\,R_A\,R_B}. \tag{10.14}$$

*Example 10.10:* Calculate the resolving time of a scintillation detector which gave 2000 counts/sec with source $A$, 4450 counts/ sec with sources $A$ and $B$, and 2500 counts/sec with source B.

$$\tau = \frac{2000 + 2500 - 4450}{2 \times 2000 \times 2500}\ \text{sec}$$

$$= \frac{50}{10 \times 10^6}\ \text{sec}$$

$$= 5\,\mu\ \text{sec.}$$

The true count rate $R_t$ will be larger than the observed count rate $R_o$ due to the dead time of the detector. The true count rate $R_t$ can be calculated knowing the resolving time $\tau$ and the observed count rate from the equation

$$R_t = \frac{R_o}{1 - R_o\tau}. \tag{10.15}$$

*Example 10.11:* Calculate the true count rates if the observed count rates are 10,000/sec and 50,000/sec when measured with a detector whose dead time is 5 $\mu$sec.

$$\text{For } R_o = 10,000,\ R_t = \frac{10,000}{1 - 10,000 \times 5 \times 10^{-6}}$$

$$= \frac{10^4}{1 - 10^4 \times 5 \times 10^{-6}}$$

$$= \frac{10^4}{1 - 5 \times 10^{-2}}$$

$$= \frac{10^4}{1 - 0.05}$$

$$= \frac{10^4}{0.95}$$

$$= 1.0526 \times 10^4$$

$$= 10,526 \text{ counts/sec.}$$

$$\text{For } R_o = 50,000, \; R_t = \frac{5 \times 10^4}{1 - 0.25}$$

$$= \frac{5 \times 10^4}{0.75} = 66,666/\text{sec.}$$

As seen from the above example, the count loss becomes significant at high count rates.

## INFORMATION DENSITY

In nuclear medicine, one is concerned with the distribution of radio-active material in the organ of interest. One of the important factors in the interpretation of tracer distribution images is the number of counts per unit area of the image, which is known as the *information* or *count density*. This factor is related to the amount of activity in the region of interest. Two other factors influencing the detectability of an abnormal area are: the size of the abnormal area and the contrast, which is the target-to-non-target count ratio. The resolution capability of the instrument used limits the minimum size of the abnormal area that can be delineated.

In principle, the statistical uncertainty becomes less as the information density increases, i.e. counting more photons carrying information on the radionuclide distribution. This might require long counting times or the administration of a higher dose of the radionuclide. The latter is limited by the absorbed dose to the patient and by the dead time of the detection in-strument. Therefore, for a given amount of administered radionuclide, higher information density means larger counting times. Thus, the informa-tion density is directly proportional to the imaging time.

Considering that the resolution capability of a scintillation detector is about 1 cm, an information density of 1000 counts/cm$^2$ is found to be satis-factory to obtain an image within a practical counting time with a reason-able statistical accuracy. Count densities less than 1000 counts/cm$^2$ can be used when the amounts administered are restricted based on dosimetric considerations.

*Example 10.12:* How many counts are needed to image a circular phantom of diameter 20 cm with an information dens-ity of 1000 counts/cm$^2$?

Area of a circle equals $\pi r^2$ where $r$ is the radius;

$$A = 3.14 \times 10^2 = 314 \; cm^2.$$

Number of counts required $= 314 \times 1000 = 314,000$ counts

The information density is, therefore, directly proportional to the administered activity, the uptake in the organ, and the thickness of the organ. Since the count rate increases as the photon attenuation decreases, the information density can be improved by using high-energy photons and thick NaI crystals.

In scanning systems, the information density is dependent on the line spacing and the speed at which the detector moves over the organ of interest. These are usually adjusted to obtain the desired information density for the given amount of administered dose and the organ uptake.

Finally, information densities greater than 1000 counts/cm² are not gainful for most diagnostic procedures with the present imaging systems. In other words, the probability of detection of a lesion with a scintillation camera does not increase very much by increasing the information density over 1000 counts/cm². When the size of the lesion is more than 2 or 3 cm diameter, an information density of 400 to 500 counts/cm² is enough to delineate the lesion.

## PROBLEMS AND QUESTIONS

1. The total number of counts collected is 2,500. The standard error is
   (A) 1 percent.
   (B) 2 percent.
   (C) 3 percent.
   (D) 4 percent.

2. The 96 percent confidence interval for 2,500 counts is
   (A) 2400 to 2600.
   (B) 2450 to 2550.
   (C) 2400 to 2550.
   (D) 2450 to 2500.

3. The number of counts required to obtain a standard error of 1 percent is
   (A) 80,000.
   (B) 40,000.
   (C) 20,000.
   (D) 10,000.

4. The background count is 400 and the sample count is 2,100. The standard deviation in the net count is
   (A) 20.
   (B) 41.
   (C) 50.
   (D) 45.

5. In the absence of background, a sample counted for 5 minutes gave

8,000 counts. The standard error is
   (A) 1.1.
   (B) 3.1.
   (C) 2.5.
   (D) 5.

6. The probable error in the count rate of the above measurement is
   (A) 40.
   (B) 27.
   (C) 12.
   (D) 50.

7. The resolving time of a counting system determines the
   (A) pulse duration.
   (B) least period of time in which an accurate count can be determined.
   (C) number of counts lost at high counting rates.
   (D) minimum counts per unit time that can be accurately determined.

8. The resolving time of a detection system is 10 $\mu$sec. What is the true count if the observed count is 10,000/sec?
   (A) 11,100.
   (B) 10,000.
   (C)  9,100.
   (D) 12,200.

9. Information density is
   (A) the total number of counts divided by scanning time.
   (B) the scanning time divided by the total counts.
   (C) the count rate per unit area.
   (D) the counts per unit area.

10. The total number of counts required to image a liver whose approximate area is 250 cm² with an information density of 800 counts/cm², are
   (A) 200,000.
   (B)  80,000.
   (C) 250,000.
   (D) 150,000.

# 11

# Radiation safety

All persons who are in any way involved in the use of radioactive materials should be aware of the possible hazards and should know the proper procedures and precautions to be taken. This is essential for two reasons: to avoid excessive and unnecessary exposure to personnel, and to avoid radioactive contamination or radiation levels which might interfere with the results of tests or studies being performed. In this chapter will be considered permissible exposure levels, radiation hazards, and proper safety procedures.

## RADIATION UNITS

The unit of radiation dosage is the *rad,* which will be further discussed in the next chapter. The rad is a unit of energy absorption, defined as an absorption of 100 ergs per gram of any material.* However, for radiation measurement purposes another and older unit is still relevant: the *roentgen* (R), which is a unit of radiation exposure. One method of accurately determining radiation exposure levels is to measure the ionization produced in air. Thus the roentgen is a unit of radiation exposure, representing essentially that amount of x or gamma radiation which will produce ionization equal to one electrostatic unit of charge per cubic centimeter of air. The relation between the roentgen and the rad depends on the photon energy and the atomic number of the material being irradiated. For low-atomic number materials, such as water, plastics and soft tissue, and for

---

*Recently the ICRU has recommended the use of the gray, symbol Gy, equal to one joule per kilogram. Thus I Gy = 100 rad = 1 J/Kg.

photon energies greater than 100 keV, the factor is about 0.95 rads/roentgen.

For specifying permissible radiation doses to personnel, another unit, the *rem,* is used. The rem was introduced to allow for the fact that some types of radiation, for example, neutrons and alpha particles, may produce more biological damage than x or gamma rays for the same physical dose. At one time the rem was defined as the rad times the RBE, or relative biological effect; more recently, in order not to make the definition dependent on any one biological system, the rem has been defined as the rad times the quality factor, Q, and any other appropriate modifying factors. The factor Q may be related to the LET, or linear energy transfer, of the radiation; for example, heavy charged particles such as protons and alpha particles which produce densely ionized paths have a high linear energy transfer and thus are assigned a high value of Q. However, for radiation having a LET of less than 3.5 keV per micron of path length, which includes most x rays, gamma rays, and electrons, the value of Q is taken as 1.0. Thus the rem is equal to the rad, and approximately equal to the roentgen, so that in nuclear medicine the three units are more or less equivalent and for protection purposes are often used interchangeably.

## RADIATION EXPOSURE LIMITS

Everyone receives a radiation dose of at least 0.1 rem per year, or an exposure level of about 100 mR/year. This is the so-called background level, resulting primarily from three sources: about 20 mR/year from $^{40}$K within the body, since $^{40}$K, a beta-gamma emitter, occurs as 0.01 percent of natural potassium; and the remainder due more or less equally to cosmic radiation and radiations from naturally occurring radioactive materials in the ground and in building materials such as brick and concrete. Doses due to the latter may vary by $\pm 50$ percent with different locations and different types of construction, while cosmic-ray levels vary with latitude and with altitude, doubling at about 5000 feet.

Thus it is impossible not to receive any radiation exposures; the question is, what is a safe exposure level for occupationally exposed persons? There is no clear-cut answer, but various recommended values for maximum permissible radiation doses (MPD) to occupationally exposed persons have been formulated by the National Council on Radiation Protection and Measurements (NCRP) and by the International Commission on Radiological Protection (ICRP). The background of how these values were determined has been presented in various publications of the NCRP and ICRP, particularly NCRP Report no. 39, *Basic Radiation Protection Criteria.* The NCRP is not a government agency, but its recommended values have been more or less adopted by the Nuclear Regulatory Commission (NRC) and also have been written into many state and local health codes, thus becoming legally enforceable.

The recommended MPD for occupationally exposed persons may be summarized as follows:

*Whole body, gonads, lens of the eye,* and *red blood marrow:* 5 rems in any one year. The NRC lists $1\frac{1}{4}$ rem/quarter; both the NRC and the NCRP allow up to 3 rem/quarter provided the average does not exceed 5 rem/year, i.e. the accumulated occupational dose to the whole body does not exceed 5 (N-18) where N is the individual's age.
*Skin* (other than hands and forearms): 15 rem/year. NRC: $7\frac{1}{2}$/quarter.
*Hands:* 75 rem/year; maximum 25 rem/quarter. NRC: $18\frac{3}{4}$/quarter.
*Forearms:* 30 rem/year; maximum 10 rem/quarter. NRC: $18\frac{3}{4}$/quarter.
*All other organs:* 15 rem/year.

The recommended limit for whole-body doses for persons not occupationally exposed is 0.5 rem/year in addition to natural background and medical and dental exposures. A further recommendation concerns the occupational exposure of a pregnant woman: The MPD to the fetus from occupational exposure to the expectant mother is 0.5 rem.

Since it is desirable to keep the dose to occupationally exposed persons below an average of 5 rem per year, the value of 5 roentgen/year or approximately 100 mR/week has generally been taken as a maximum permissible exposure level for occupied areas. This value, although not stated by the NCRP, has nevertheless been adopted by the NRC and many health codes. Thus radiation shielding around radioactive sources should be designed to reduce the exposure levels to less than 100 mR/week for areas that might be occupied by nuclear medicine personnel. Areas where the occupational exposure of personnel is under the control of the radiation protection supervisor are known as controlled areas. Areas occupied by persons whose radiation doses are not monitored are known as noncontrolled areas. Maximum permissible exposure levels to noncontrolled areas are generally taken as 10 mR/week.

## RADIATION HAZARDS

In general there are two types of hazards associated with the use of radioactive materials in nuclear medicine: gamma-ray exposures from unshielded or inadequately shielded sources, and contamination resulting from accidental spills or leaks of radioactive solutions. The first type may lead to personnel receiving exposures in excess of those given in the previous section, while contamination may interfere with future tests and procedures, as well as present a hazard to personnel. Methods of avoiding contamination will be discussed later, but first protection from gamma-emitting radionuclides will be considered.

## GAMMA-RAY PROTECTION

The gamma-ray output of a radionuclide may be specified in terms of a constant, sometimes known as the gamma factor, the specific gamma-ray constant, or the exposure rate constant, with the symbol that of a capital gamma: $\Gamma$. Several combinations of units have been used, but the preferred ones are roentgens per hour per millicurie at one centimeter, sometimes written R-cm$^2$/mCi-hr. The definitive of $\Gamma$ should include all photons, both gamma rays and characteristic X rays, but for protection purposes only photons greater than about 20 keV need be included, as photons with less than 20 keV energy will normally be absorbed by any source container. The values of $\Gamma$ for a few commonly used radionuclides are given in Table 11-I. An example of the use of the gamma factor will now be given.

> *Example 11.1:* Prior to injecting a patient, 15 millicuries of $^{99m}$Tc are drawn into a syringe. What is the exposure rate to a person standing about 50 cm from the syringe?
>
> From table 11-I, the exposure rate for $^{99m}$Tc is 0.6. Since the output from a point source varies inversely as the square of the distance, the amount of exposure is divided by the square of the distance in cm:

$$\frac{0.6 \ R\text{-}cm^2/mCi\text{-}hr \times 15 \ mCi}{(50 \ cm)^2} = 0.0036 \ R/hr = 3.6 \ mR/hr.$$

Adequate gamma-ray protection may be achieved by either distance or shielding, or a combination of both. Any high-atomic number material may be used for shielding; but from the standpoint of cost and convenience, lead is the most suitable. The absorption in lead may be expressed in terms of the half-value layer, HVL, as discussed in Chapter 4. However, in protection problems, reductions by more than a factor of two are usually required, so that a useful concept is that of the tenth-value layer, TVL, which is the thickness required to reduce the intensity to one-tenth its original value. For single-energy photons, the TVL is equal to 3.3 HVL. Also, a reduction to 1 percent may be achieved by only 2 TVL. Some values for TVL are given in Table 11-I. Their use will now be illustrated.

> *Example.11.2:* How much lead must surround a 200 mCi $^{99}$Mo-$^{99m}$Tc generator so that the exposure rate is less than 2 mR/hr at 1 meter?
>
> Problems of this sort should be solved in two steps:
> (1) Find the output without shielding;

TABLE 11-I

GAMMA RAY PROPERTIES OF SOME RADIONUCLIDES USEFUL IN
NUCLEAR MEDICINE

| | *Principal*<br>*γ or X rays,*<br>*MeV* | $\Gamma_{20}$*<br>*R/mCi-hr*<br>*at 1 cm* | *HVL*<br>*lead*<br>*cm* | *TVL*<br>*lead*<br>*cm* |
|---|---|---|---|---|
| [51]Cr | 0.320 | 0.18 | 0.17 | 0.5 |
| [57]Co | 0.122 | 0.58 | 0.02 | 0.7 |
| [60]Co | 1.173,  1.332 | 12.96 | 1.2 | 3.8 |
| [67]Ga | 0.091-0.394 | 0.80 | 0.1 | 0.7 |
| [75]Se | 0.097-0.400 | 1.91 | 0.2 | 0.8 |
| [99]Mo | 0.140-0.778 | 1.45 | 0.7 | 2.1 |
| [99m]Tc | 0.140 | 0.60 | 0.03 | 0.8 |
| [123]I | 0.027,  0.159 | 1.53 | 0.04 | 1.2 |
| [125]I | 0.027-0.035 | 1.41 | 0.002 | 0.01 |
| [131]I | 0.364,  0.637 | 2.16 | 0.3 | 1.7 |
| [127]Xe | 0.028-0.375 | 2.15 | 0.002 | 0.01 |
| [133]Xe | 0.031,  0.081 | 0.51 | 0.03 | 0.09 |
| [165]Er | 0.047,  0.054 | 0.31 | 0.007 | 0.02 |
| [197]Hg | 0.068,  0.077 | 0.36 | 0.03 | 0.1 |

*$\Gamma_{20}$ = Exposure rate constant for all photons greater than 20 keV. Calculated from data in Dillman, L. T. and Von der Lage, F. C., MIRD Pamphlet No. 10, New York, Society of Nuclear Medicine, 1975.

(2) Use the HVL or TVL concept to reduce the output to the desired value.

*Step 1:* From table 11-I, $\Gamma = 1.45$. Thus at 1 meter,

$$\frac{1.45 \times 200 \, mCi}{(100 \, cm)^2} = 0.029 \, R/hr = 29 \, mR/hr.$$

*Step 2:* From table 11-I,

One *TVL* (2.1 *cm*) reduces the exposure to 2.9 *mR/hr*. An additional *HVL* (0.7 *cm*) reduces to 1.5 *mR/hr*.

Thus about 2.8 cm, or slightly more than 1 inch, is required to reduce the exposure rate to less than 2 mR/hr at 1 meter.

With low-energy gamma emitters, even small amounts of lead may be useful. For example, with [99m]Tc, a lead apron of the type used in diagnostic radiology having a lead equivalent of 0.5 mm will reduce the exposure to about one third of the unshielded value.

## LABORATORY PRECAUTIONS

Avoiding contamination when working with radioactive solutions requires proper equipment, adequate space, and carefully planned procedures. Anyone transferring solutions from one container to another should wear plastic gloves and use trays covered with absorbent paper. In case of accidental spills, absorbent paper should be placed on the spill, the area blocked off, and the radiation safety officer notified.

Any areas where radioactive solutions are prepared or injected should be checked daily using a portable survey meter, as described in the next section. Used syringes and empty bottles should be placed in a marked container, which may require a small amount of shielding. Radioactive sources with no further use should be stored in shielded areas for about ten half-lives and then placed in a marked container, which should be periodically collected by a commercial service. Other radioactive waste can be disposed of in this way. In general, radioactive solutions should not be dumped "down the sink." Although disposing of small amounts by this route may be permissible, the amount depends on the radionuclide and the dilution factor, i.e. the water flow from the entire hospital. For most nuclides and typical hospital discharge volumes, this works out to less than 10 $\mu$Ci per day. Thus for nuclear medicine departments, where the amounts involved may be millicuries or at least hundreds of microcuries, disposal by the sink is to be avoided.

## RADIATION-MONITORING INSTRUMENTS

The principles of radiation detection with air and gas-filled detectors were presented in Chapter 8. Here will be mentioned several types of instruments which are used for radiation monitoring and radiation protection measurements in a nuclear medicine department or lab using radionuclides, and their usefulness and limitations will be discussed.

Geiger-type Survey Meter. The most useful instrument for a nuclear medicine department is a simple portable Geiger survey meter, as shown in Figure 11-1. Typically the Geiger tube is a thin-walled cylinder mounted in a metal tube, so that it is intended primarily for gamma-ray detection. In some cases part of the metal sleeve may be removed, allowing for detection of high-energy beta particles, such as those from $^{32}$P. The individual pulses may be amplified to produce clicks in a loudspeaker, and also fed to a rate meter, which shows the approximate number of counts per second or per minute. The meter may also be labeled "mR/hr," although this may be only approximately correct. A Geiger counter only counts events; it does not measure roentgens, which are based on the measurement of ionization in air. However, the meter may be calibrated in mR/hr by using a gamma source, such as $^{137}$Cs or $^{60}$Co, whose activity and gamma factor are accurately known. The meter will then read correctly for high-energy gamma rays but may be off by 50 percent or more for other energies.

Another type of instrument using a Geiger tube is an area radiation monitor, of the type widely used in high-activity laboratories. A high rate

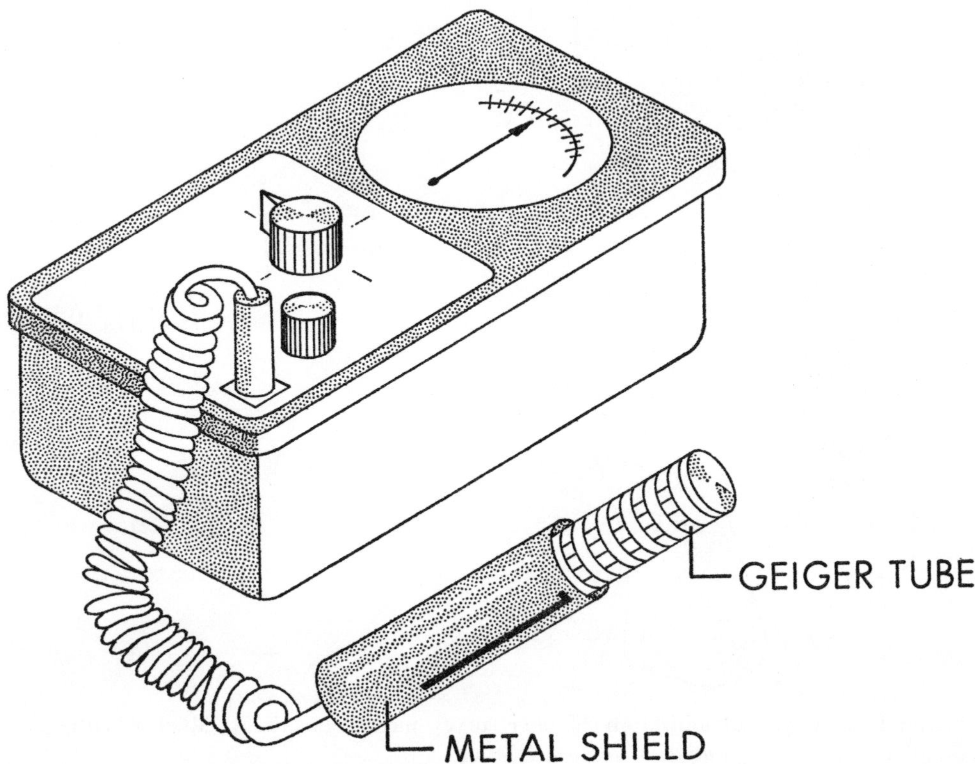


Figure 11-1. A typical Geiger-type survey meter, useful for detecting radiation hazards or contamination due to gamma-emitting radionuclides.

of pulses from the detector, which is usually a Geiger tube, may trigger a relay which turns on a red light or produces an audible warning when a predetermined radiation level is exceeded.

Geiger survey meters offer a sensitive and reliable means of determining the presence of radiation hazards or radioactive contamination. They are not suitable for measuring very high intensities, nor for accurately measuring radiation exposure levels. For these purposes an ionization-type instrument is usually required.

IONIZATION SURVEY METERS. The production of ionization in air has long been a simple and reliable means of detecting radiation and accurately determining the exposure levels involved. Consequently a large variety of ionization-type radiation monitoring instruments are available, capable of measuring exposure levels from a few mR/hr to thousands of R/min. The sensitivity of an ionization chamber is proportional to the size of the air volume from which ions are collected. Thus, to measure low levels of radiation, a fairly large ionization chamber is required.

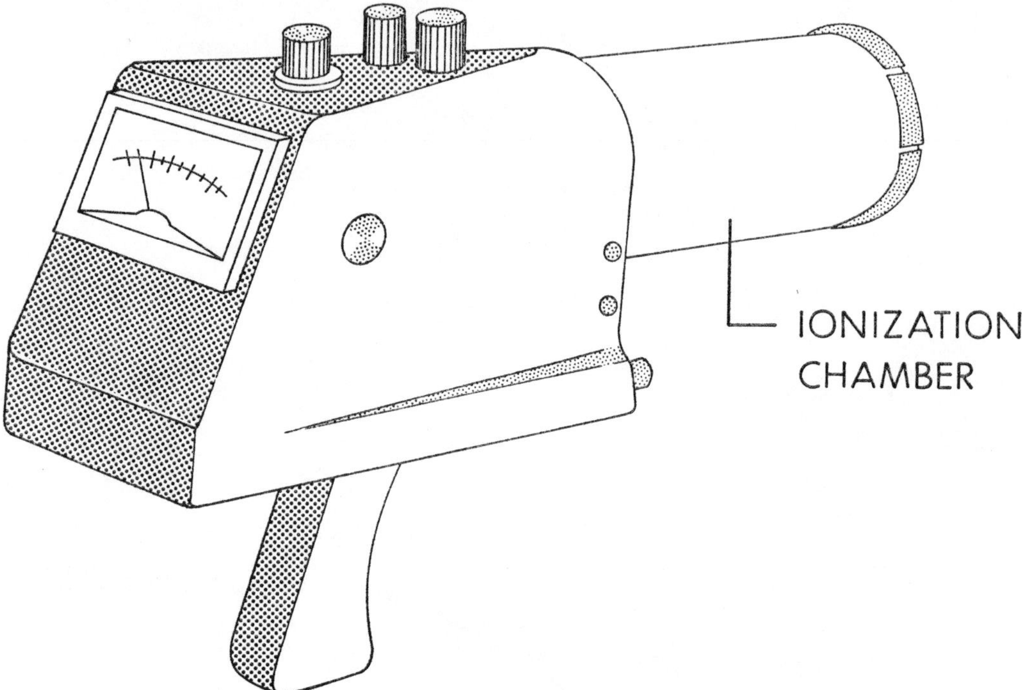


Figure 11-2. A type of ionization-chamber survey meter, sometimes called a "cutie-pie," useful for measuring radiation exposure levels.

One type of ionization survey meter which is widely used for making low-level measurements is shown in Figure 11-2. This style is commonly known as a "cutie-pie" survey meter, for reasons which are still being disputed. The ionization chamber is a cylinder about four inches in diameter and five inches long, with a central pin as the collecting electrode, and is attached directly to the instrument. Such an instrument is capable of measuring radiation levels over a wide range, from about 1 mR/hr to hundreds of R/hr.

An ionization survey meter is not as sensitive as a Geiger survey meter, but is more suitable when accurate radiation exposure levels must be determined.

## QUESTIONS AND PROBLEMS

1. The unit of radiation exposure is the
    (A) rad.
    (B) roentgen.
    (C) rem.
    (D) MPD.

2. The rad is a unit of
   (A) radiation exposure.
   (B) radiation dose.
   (C) radiation quality.
   (D) linear energy transfer.
3. The rem is defined as:
   (A) the rad times the RBE.
   (B) the roentgen times the LET.
   (C) the rad times the quality factor.
   (D) the rads per roentgen.
4. The background radiation level is about
   (A) 1 mR/year.
   (B) 10 mR/year.
   (C) 100 mR/year.
   (D) 1 R/year.
5. The MPD for occupationally exposed persons is
   (A) 3 rem/quarter.
   (B) 100 mR/week.
   (C) 3 rem/year.
   (D) 5 rem/year.
6. The MPD of a fetus from occupational exposure to the mother is
   (A) 15 rem/year.
   (B) 3 rem/quarter.
   (C) 5 rem/year.
   (D) 0.5 rem/year.
7. The exposure at a distance, $d$, from a source is proportional to
   (A) $d$.
   (B) $d^2$.
   (C) $\dfrac{1}{d}$.
   (D) $\dfrac{1}{d^2}$.
8. The exposure rate to a person 50 cm from 10 mCi of $^{131}$I is
   (A) 36 mR/hr.
   (B) 21.7 mR/hr.
   (C) 8.6 mR/hr.
   (D) 6 mR/hr.
9. The amount of lead needed to reduce the above exposure level to 2 mR/hr is about
   (A) 1 mm.
   (B) 1 cm.

(C)  2.5 cm.
(D)  10 cm.

10. Accurate measurements of radiation exposure levels can be made with
    (A)  a Geiger-counter.
    (B)  an ionization survey meter.
    (C)  both.
    (D)  neither.

11. In case of a radiation accident
    (A)  clean the area immediately.
    (B)  block the area until the source decays.
    (C)  block the area and call the radiation safety officer.
    (D)  flood the area with water.

# 12

# Radiation dosimetry

The administration of radiopharmaceuticals results in the absorption of radiation and therefore energy by the patient, causing injury to the cells by altering the molecular structure. Although the extent of injury depends on the amount of energy absorbed, all ionizing radiations are considered as harmful in general to living matter. It is therefore necessary to evaluate the potential risk to the patient before radioactive materials are administered.

The amount of energy imparted to living matter is known as the absorbed dose. The unit of absorbed dose is the *rad,* defined as 100 ergs per gram of matter.* Since an erg is equal to $6.24 \times 10^5$ MeV, the absorbed dose is one rad when a gram of matter receives $6.24 \times 10^7$ MeV of energy. The absorbed dose to an organ is determined by dividing the energy given to the matter in that organ by the mass of the organ.

The absorbed dose in nuclear medicine depends on several factors:

(1) the biological properties of the radiopharmaceutical,
(2) the physical properties of the radionuclide,
(3) the interaction properties of the radiations emitted by the radionuclide.

The lack of reliable data on the biological behavior of the radiopharmaceutical makes accurate absorbed dose calculations difficult. In this chapter will be discussed the *method of absorbed fractions* to estimate the dose. The reader is referred to the pamphlets written by the Medical Internal Radiation Dose (MIRD) Committee of the Society of Nuclear Medicine and pub-

---

*Recently the ICRU has recommended the use of the gray symbol Gy, equal to one joule per kilogram. Thus 1 Gy = 100 rad = 1 J/Kg.

lished as supplements to the *Journal of Nuclear Medicine* for more details of this method and for other useful data to calculate radiation doses.

## CUMULATIVE CONCENTRATION

The energy absorbed by an organ obviously increases with increasing uptake of the administered radiopharmaceutical, which is usually assumed to be distributed uniformly throughout the organ. Hence the average absorbed dose $(\bar{D})$ is directly proportional to the number of radioactive atoms present per gram of organ tissue, known as the *cumulative concentration* $(\tilde{C})$:

$$\bar{D} \, \alpha \, \tilde{C} = N/m, \tag{12.1}$$

where $N$ is the total number of radioactive atoms in the organ and $m$ is the mass of the organ. The number of atoms, $N$, can be calculated knowing the activity of the radionuclide in the organ. The activity $(A)$ is proportional to the total number of radioactive atoms, $N$. The proportionality constant is $\lambda$, which is equal to $\dfrac{0.693}{T_p}$ where $T_p$ is the physical half-life of the radionuclide. Mathematically,

$$A = N\lambda$$
$$A = \frac{0.693 \, N}{T_p};$$

therefore,

$$N = 1.44 \, T_p \, A. \tag{12.2}$$

Substituting for $N$ in equation (12.1),

$$\bar{D} \, \alpha \, \tilde{C} = 1.44 \, T_p \, A/m. \tag{12.3}$$

It can be seen from the above equation that the average absorbed dose increases with the physical half-life $T_p$ and the maximum organ activity $A$ and decreases with the mass of the organ. The advantage of short-lived radionuclides is now apparent.

The factor $1/\lambda$ or $1.44 \, T_p$ is known as the *average* or the *mean life* of the radionuclide. This is the time which a radionuclide decaying at a constant rate equal to its initial rate would require to produce the same number of disintegrations as a source decaying exponentially.

*Example 12.1:* Calculate the mean life of technetium-99m.

$$\text{Mean life} = 1.44 \, T_p$$
$$T_p = 6 \text{ hrs}$$
$$\text{Mean life} = 1.44 \times 6 \text{ hrs}$$
$$= 8.64 \text{ hrs}$$

This means that if a source of $^{99m}\text{Tc}$ decayed at a constant rate equal to its initial rate for 8.64 hours, it would result in the same number of disintegration as a source which decays exponentially with a half-life of 6 hours.

*Example 12.2:* About 10 mCi of $^{99m}$Tc-pharmaceutical is administered to a patient. The uptake in the liver is known to be 70 percent. Calculate the cumulative concentration $(\tilde{C})$ in the liver if the mass is 1800 gms.

$$\text{The activity in the liver} = 70\% \text{ of } 10 \; mCi$$
$$= 7 \; mCi = 7 \times 10^3 \; \mu Ci$$
$$\tilde{C} = \frac{1.44 \, T_p \, A}{m} = \frac{1.44 \times 6 \times (7 \times 10^3)}{1.8 \times 10^3} \; \frac{\mu Ci\text{-}hr}{gm}$$

$$\tilde{C} = 33.6 \; \frac{\mu Ci\text{-}hr}{gm}$$

BIOLOGIC AND EFFECTIVE HALF-LIFE. So far it has been assumed that maximum uptake of the pharmaceutical is instantaneous and that the activity $A$ in the organ is unchanged indefinitely. Maximum activity in the organ of interest is usually obtained some time after the administration of the radionuclide. Once the maximum is reached, the activity slowly decreases depending on the biological behavior of the pharmaceutical, that is, the radioactive atoms are continuously removed from the organ by biological processes. As a result, cumulative concentration in the organ and hence the absorbed dose will be less.

The *biological half-life* $T_b$ is the time taken by the system to reduce the maximum activity in the organ to half by the biological elimination process. Then the effective half-life $T_{eff}$ is the time required to reduce the initial maximum activity to half by both the biological and physical decay of the radionuclide. Since $\lambda_{eff} = \lambda_p + \lambda_b$, where $\lambda_p$ and $\lambda_b$ are physical and biological decay constants respectively, the effective half-life can be obtained by substituting for $\lambda$ in terms of half-lives as

$$\frac{1}{T_{eff}} = \frac{1}{T_p} + \frac{1}{T_b} \text{, or } T_{eff} = \frac{T_b \times T_p}{T_b + T_p}. \qquad (12.4)$$

If $T_p$ is much larger than $T_b$, the biological half-life $T_b$ can be neglected in the denominator of equation (12.4). Then

$$T_{eff} = T_b \text{ if } T_p \gg T_b.$$

Similarly,

$$T_{eff} = T_p \text{ if } T_b \gg T_p.$$

The cumulative concentration $\tilde{C}$ can be obtained by substituting $T_{eff}$ for $T_p$ in equation (12.3):

$$\tilde{C} = \frac{1.44 \, A}{m} \, T_{eff}. \qquad (12.5)$$

The assumption that the uptake of radionuclide by the organ is instantaneous overestimates the cumulative concentration and hence the absorbed dose. This is particularly so when the biological half-time for uptake, $T_{bu}$ is comparable to the physical half-life of the radionuclide. When short-lived isotopes are involved, the time required for uptake $(T_{up})$ should be considered. The cumulative concentration $\tilde{C}$ can be calculated from

$$\tilde{C} = \frac{1.44\,A}{m}\,T_{eff}\left(1 - \frac{T_{up}}{T_{eff}}\right),\qquad(12.6)$$

where

$$T_{up} = \frac{T_p \times T_{bu}}{T_p + T_{bu}},$$

and $A$ is projected activity at $t = 0$.

Note that when $T_{up}$ is very small compared to $T_{eff}$, equation (12.6) reduces to equation (12.5). The biological half-life and the uptake half-time can be obtained by taking samples of the tissue and counting for the activity at different times after the administration of the radionuclide and by plotting the activity versus time. Biological distribution studies are obviously difficult in humans and are usually supplemented by studies in experimental animals.

The biological half-life may not be the same for all organs and may contain more than one component, in which case the cumulative concentration should be summed over all components. When the biological half-life and the uptake half-time are not known, the effective half-life is taken as equal to the physical half-life and the uptake is assumed to be instantaneous. It is always safer to overestimate the dose than to underestimate.

*Example 12.3:* Calculate the $T_{eff}$ if the biological half-life of a $^{99m}$Tc pharmaceutical in the organ is (1) 0.5 hrs, (2) 10 hrs, (3) 6 days.

For $^{99m}$Tc, $T_p$ is 6 hours.

(1) $T_b = 0.5$ hrs;

$$T_{eff} = \frac{6 \times 0.5}{6 + 0.5} = \frac{3}{6.5} = 0.46 \text{ hrs.}$$

(2) $T_b = 10$ hrs;

$$T_{eff} = \frac{6 \times 10}{6 + 10} = \frac{60}{16} = 3.75 \text{ hrs.}$$

(3) $T_b = 6$ days;

$$T_{eff} = \frac{6 \times 6 \times 24}{6 + 6 \times 24} = \frac{864}{150} = 5.8 \text{ hrs.}$$

*Example 12.4:* Calculate the cumulative concentration of a $^{99m}$Tc pharmaceutical in the liver if: (1) $T_b = 6$ days, $T_{bu} = 0.01$ hrs; (2) $T_b = 6$ days, $T_{bu} = 1$ hr. The administered dose is 10 mCi and the maximum liver uptake is 70 percent.

(1) $T_b = 6$ days; $T_{eff} = 5.8$ hrs from the previous example.

$$T_{bu} = 0.01 \text{ hrs}; \quad T_{up} = \frac{T_u \times T_{bu}}{T_u + T_{bu}} = \frac{6 \times 0.01}{6 + 0.01} = \frac{0.06}{6.01} = 0.01 \text{ hrs.}$$

$$\tilde{C} = \frac{1.44\,A}{m}\, T_{eff} \left( 1 - \frac{T_{up}}{T_{eff}} \right)$$

$$\tilde{C} = \frac{1.44 \times 7 \times 10^3}{1.8 \times 10^3} \times 5.8 \left( 1 - \frac{0.01}{5.8} \right)\, \frac{\mu Ci\text{-}hr}{gm}$$

$$= 32.5\, \frac{\mu Ci\text{-}hr}{gm}$$

Since $T_{bu}$ is much less than $T_{eff}$, the same result will be obtained by using equation (12.5).

(2) $T_b = 6$ days; $T_{eff} = 5.8$ hrs;

$$T_{bu} = 1 \text{ hr}; \quad T_{up} = \frac{6 \times 1}{6 + 1} = \frac{6}{7} = 0.86 \text{ hrs.}$$

$$\tilde{C} = \frac{1.44 \times 7 \times 10^3}{1.8 \times 10^3} \times 5.8 \left( 1 - \frac{0.86}{5.8} \right)\, \frac{\mu Ci\text{-}hr}{gm}$$

$$= 32.5 \times (1 - 0.15)\, \frac{\mu Ci\text{-}hr}{gm}$$

$$= 32.5 \times 0.85\, \frac{\mu Ci\text{-}hr}{gm}$$

$$= 27.6\, \frac{\mu Ci\text{-}hr}{gm}$$

## EQUILIBRIUM ABSORBED DOSE CONSTANT

The energy absorbed by an organ is also proportional to the energy of the radiation emitted by the radionuclide. Each disintegration might result in the emission of one or more radiations. All these radiations should be considered. The *equilibrium absorbed dose constant,* denoted by the symbol $\Delta$, is the total energy released by the radionuclide per disintegration. It is equal to the sum of the individual equilibrium absorbed dose constants, which are each given by

$$\Delta_i = N_i E_i \ MeV/dis.$$

where $\Delta_i$ is the equilibrium absorbed dose constant, $N_i$ is the fractional frequency and $E_i$ is the energy in $MeV$ of the particular type of radiation $(i)$.

The equilibrium absorbed dose constant can be expressed in more convenient units.

$$MeV/dis. = 1.6 \times 10^{-6} \times 10^{-2} \frac{rads\text{-}gm}{ergs} \times \frac{3.7 \times 10^4}{\mu Ci - sec} \times 3600 \frac{sec}{hr}$$

$$= 2.13 \frac{gm\text{-}rads}{\mu Ci\text{-hr}}$$

Then, the equilibrium absorbed dose constant

$$\Delta_i = 2.13 \, N_i E_i \frac{gm\text{-}rads}{\mu Ci\text{-hr}}. \tag{12.7}$$

The equilibrium absorbed dose constants for all radiations are given in the "Supplements" to *The Journal of Nuclear Medicine* for all useful radionuclides. For beta rays, the average energy is used to calculate these constants.

*Example 12.5:* Assuming the emission of one 140 keV photon each time a $^{99m}$Tc atom disintegrates, calculate the equilibrium absorbed dose constant.

Since each disintegration results in the emission of a 140 keV photon, $N_i = 1$, $E_i = 0.14$ MeV.

$$\Delta_i = 2.13 \times 1 \times 0.14 \frac{gm\text{-}rads}{\mu Ci\text{-hr}}$$

$$= 0.30 \frac{gm\text{-}rads}{\mu Ci\text{-hr}}$$

*Example 12.6:* Calculate the equilibrium absorbed dose constant if the radionuclide disintegrates by the emission of a positron only with a maximum energy of 1.5 MeV.

For a positron, $N_i = 1$;

Average energy, $E_i = \dfrac{E_{max}}{3} = 0.5$ MeV.

$$\Delta_i = 2.13 \times 1 \times 0.5 = 1.06 \frac{gm\text{-}rad}{\mu Ci\text{-hr}}.$$

A positron eventually annihilates with an electron giving two photons of energy 0.511 MeV each. Therefore, for the photons, $N_i = 2$; $E_i = 0.511$ MeV.

$$\Delta_i = 2.13 \times 2 \times 0.511 \frac{gm\text{-}rad}{\mu Ci\text{-hr}}$$

$$= 2.18 \frac{gm\text{-}rad}{\mu Ci\text{-hr}}.$$

The total energy per disintegration

$$\Delta = (\Delta_i) \text{ positron} + (\Delta_i) \text{ gamma}$$

$$= 1.06 + 2.18 = 3.24 \frac{gm\text{-}rad}{\mu Ci\text{-hr}}.$$

## ABSORBED FRACTION

So far discussed has been the number of radioactive atoms present per gram of tissue, $\tilde{C}$, and the energy emitted by the radionuclide, $\Delta$. It is also necessary to know the fraction of the energy absorbed by the organ to complete the dose calculation. The absorbed fraction of the energy depends on the kind and energy of the radiations. Nonpenetrating radiations such as electrons and photons of energy less than 10 keV are absorbed by the organ from which they originate. In case of penetrating photons, a fraction of the energy is absorbed by the source organ and a small fraction by the nearby organs. For example, the radiation emitted from the liver imparts some energy to the spleen, lungs, kidneys, etc.

The organ in which the absorbed dose is being calculated is the *target organ*. Ideally, one needs to consider not only the absorbed fraction due to the target activity, but also the absorbed fraction due to the activity in the nontarget tissue. This makes the calculation more complicated.

The absorbed fraction $(\Phi_i)$ is defined as the energy deposited in the target tissue by the particular type of radiation $(i)$ emitted by the radionuclide in the source tissue divided by the energy of the particular type of radiation $(i)$ emitted by the radionuclide in the source tissue.

$$\Phi_i = \frac{E_i \text{ (deposited)}}{E_i \text{ (emitted)}}$$

Since the absorbed fraction is a function of the energy and of the kind of radiation, it must be computed for each of the radiations emitted by the radionuclide. The absorbed fraction for nonpenetrating radiations is 1 for target-to-target photons, and 0 for non-target to-target photons. The absorbed fractions for penetrating radiations of uniform distribution in the source tissue are tabulated in pamphlet No. 5 of the *Journal of Nuclear Medicine Supplement 3*. The masses of several organs of a 70 kg standard-weight patient and the target-to-target absorbed fractions for photons of 140 keV energy are given in Table 12-I.

## AVERAGE ABSORBED DOSE

The equation for the average absorbed dose calculation can now be given as

$$\bar{D} = \tilde{C} \, \Sigma \, \Delta_i \, \Phi_i \tag{12.8}$$

The product $\Delta_i \, \Phi_i$ should be summed over for all the radiation emitted by the radionuclide. For nonpenetrating radiation, the above equation reduces to

$$\bar{D}_{np} = \tilde{C} \, \Sigma \, \Delta_i = \tilde{C} \, \Delta. \tag{12.9}$$

TABLE 12-I

**MASS OF ORGANS AND ABSORBED FRACTIONS FOR 140 keV PHOTONS**

| Organ Containing Uniform Source | Mass (gm) | Absorbed Fraction for 140 keV Photons Target to Target |
|---|---|---|
| Total body | 70,000 | 0.35 |
| Bladder | 500 | 0.117 |
| Kidneys | 290 | 0.067 |
| Liver | 1,800 | 0.162 |
| Lungs | 1,000 | 0.049 |
| Pancreas | 60 | 0.04 |
| Skeleton | 10,000 | 0.153 |
| Spleen | 175 | 0.072 |
| Thyroid | 20 | 0.029 |
| Brain | 1,470 | 0.16 |

The average absorbed dose should be calculated for the organs that are irradiated for the longest time or have a high concentration of the radionuclide.

When the biological half-life and uptake half-time are not available, the physical half-life should be taken as the effective half-life and instantaneous uptake is assumed. The dose to the critical organ, the organ receiving the highest dose, should be calculated. The dose to the gonads should be calculated always. If the concentration of activity in the gonads is not known, it should be assumed to be the same as the blood concentration.

The average absorbed dose for $^{99m}$Tc-pharmaceuticals can be written as

$$\bar{D} = 8.64 \frac{A}{m} (0.26\,\Phi + 0.04)\ rads \tag{12.10}$$

In obtaining the above equation, it is assumed the uptake is instantaneous and $T_{eff}$ is equal to $T_p$; $A$ is the activity present in the target organ; $m$ is the mass of the target organ; and $\Phi$ is the target-to-target absorbed fraction, given in Table 12-I for several organs. The dose to the target organ from the activity in the nontarget organs is not included in the above equation. This equation is useful to calculate and compare the dose to an organ from different $^{99m}$Tc-pharmaceuticals.

*Example 12.7:* Calculate the average absorbed dose to the whole body assuming uniform distribution of 10 mCi of $^{99m}$Tc-compound and no biological excretion.

$$m = 70,000\ gms$$
$$\Phi = 0.35$$
$$\bar{D} = 8.64 \frac{10 \times 10^3}{70 \times 10^3} (0.26 \times 0.35 + 0.04)$$
$$= 0.16\ rads$$

## QUESTIONS AND PROBLEMS

1. A sample of tissue weighing 2 gm received 2 rads of dose. The energy absorbed per gram of tissue is
   (A) 200 ergs.
   (B) 100 ergs.
   (C) 400 ergs.
   (D) 50 ergs.

2. The cumulative concentration is
   (A) directly proportional to the mass of the organ.
   (B) directly proportional to the square of the mass of the organ.
   (C) inversely proportional to the mass of the organ.
   (D) inversely proportional to the square of the mass of the organ.

3. The mean-life of $^{131}$I is
   (A) 8 days.
   (B) 5.5 days.
   (C) 6 hours.
   (D) 11.5 days.

4. The biological half-life of $^{131}$I in a thyroid is found to be 5 days. The effective half-life is
   (A) 8 days.
   (B) 5 days.
   (C) 11.5 days.
   (D) 3 days.

5. The radionuclide phosphorus-32 emits electrons of average energy 0.7 MeV. The absorbed dose constant is
   (A) $15 \frac{\text{gm-rad}}{\mu\text{Ci-hr}}$.
   (B) 2.13.
   (C) 0.7.
   (D) 1.5.

6. The absorbed fraction depends on the
   (A) kind of the radiation only.
   (B) energy of the radiation only.
   (C) kind and energy of the radiation.
   (D) absorbed dose constant only.

7. A source emitting 140 keV beta particles is distributed uniformly in the brain. The brain-absorbed fraction is
   (A) 0.
   (B) 1.
   (C) 0.16.
   (D) 0.14.

8. The average absorbed dose to an organ will be overestimated if it is assumed that
   (A) the radionuclide emits only one photon.
   (B) the source is uniformly distributed.
   (C) the effective half-life is equal to the physical half-life.
   (D) the uptake is not instantaneous.

9. The absorbed dose to an organ is ________ with beta particles when compared to photons of the same energy if the other parameters of the radionuclide and the distribution are the same.
   (A) less
   (B) more
   (C) same
   (D) twice

10. The average absorbed dose cannot be calculated accurately mainly because
   (A) physical properties of the radionuclides are not known completely.
   (B) the absorbed fraction is difficult to calculate.
   (C) biological distribution data is hard to obtain.
   (D) absorbed dose constants are not precise.

# Appendix I

## ALPHABETIC LIST OF THE ELEMENTS

| Element | Symbol | Atomic number Z |
|---|---|---|
| Actinium | Ac | 89 |
| Aluminum | Al | 13 |
| Americium | Am | 95 |
| Antimony | Sb | 51 |
| Argon | Ar | 18 |
| Arsenic | As | 33 |
| Astatine | At | 85 |
| Barium | Ba | 56 |
| Berkelium | Bk | 97 |
| Beryllium | Be | 4 |
| Bismuth | Bi | 83 |
| Boron | B | 5 |
| Bromine | Br | 35 |
| Cadmium | Cd | 48 |
| Calcium | Ca | 20 |
| Californium | Cf | 98 |
| Carbon | C | 6 |
| Cerium | Ce | 58 |
| Cesium | Cs | 55 |
| Chlorine | Cl | 17 |
| Chromium | Cr | 24 |

| Element | Symbol | Atomic number Z |
|---|---|---|
| Cobalt | Co | 27 |
| Copper | Cu | 29 |
| Curium | Cm | 96 |
| Dysprosium | Dy | 66 |
| Einsteinium | E | 99 |
| Erbium | Er | 68 |
| Europium | Eu | 63 |
| Fermium | Fm | 100 |
| Fluorine | F | 9 |
| Francium | Fr | 87 |
| Gadolinium | Gd | 64 |
| Gallium | Ga | 31 |
| Germanium | Ge | 32 |
| Gold | Au | 79 |
| Hafnium | Hf | 72 |
| Helium | He | 2 |
| Holmium | Ho | 67 |
| Hydrogen | H | 1 |
| Indium | In | 49 |
| Iodine | I | 53 |
| Iridium | Ir | 77 |
| Iron | Fe | 26 |
| Krypton | Kr | 36 |
| Lanthanum | La | 57 |
| Lead | Pb | 82 |
| Lithium | Li | 3 |
| Lutetium | Lu | 71 |
| Magnesium | Mg | 12 |
| Manganese | Mn | 25 |
| Mendelevium | Md | 101 |
| Mercury | Hg | 80 |
| Molybdenum | Mo | 42 |
| Neodymium | Nd | 60 |
| Neon | Ne | 10 |
| Neptunium | Np | 93 |
| Nickel | Ni | 28 |
| Niobium | Nb | 41 |
| Nitrogen | N | 7 |

| Element | Symbol | Atomic number Z |
|---|---|---|
| Nobelium | No | 102 |
| Osmium | Os | 76 |
| Oxygen | O | 8 |
| Palladium | Pd | 46 |
| Phosphorus | P | 15 |
| Platinum | Pt | 78 |
| Plutonium | Pu | 94 |
| Polonium | Po | 84 |
| Potassium | K | 19 |
| Prascodymium | Pr | 59 |
| Promethium | Pm | 61 |
| Protactinium | Pa | 91 |
| Radium | Ra | 88 |
| Radon | Rn | 86 |
| Rhenium | Re | 75 |
| Rhodium | Rh | 45 |
| Rubidium | Rb | 37 |
| Ruthenium | Ru | 44 |
| Samarium | Sm | 62 |
| Scandium | Sc | 21 |
| Selenium | Se | 34 |
| Silicon | Si | 14 |
| Silver | Ag | 47 |
| Sodium | Na | 11 |
| Strontium | Sr | 38 |
| Sulfur | S | 16 |
| Tantalum | Ta | 73 |
| Technetium | Tc | 43 |
| Tellurium | Te | 52 |
| Terbium | Tb | 65 |
| Thallium | Tl | 81 |
| Thorium | Th | 90 |
| Thulium | Tm | 69 |
| Tin | Sn | 50 |
| Titanium | Ti | 22 |
| Tungsten | W | 74 |
| Uranium | U | 92 |
| Vanadium | V | 23 |

| Element | Symbol | Atomic number Z |
|---|---|---|
| Xenon | Xe | 54 |
| Ytterbium | Yb | 70 |
| Yttrium | Y | 39 |
| Zinc | Zn | 30 |
| Zirconium | Zr | 40 |

# Appendix II



**CONVERSION FACTORS**

1 becquerel (Bq) $= 1$ dis/sec

1 curie (Ci) $= 3.7 \times 10^{10}$ dis/sec $= 37$ GBq

1 millicurie (mCi) $= 3.7 \times 10^{7}$ dis/sec $= 37$ MBq

1 microcurie ($\mu$Ci) $= 3.7 \times 10^{4}$ dis/sec $= 37$ kBq

1 nanocurie (nCi) $= 37$ dis/sec $= 37$ Bq

1 eV $= 1.602 \times 10^{-12}$ ergs

1 keV $= 1.602 \times 10^{-9}$ ergs

1 MeV $= 1.602 \times 10^{-6}$ ergs

1 erg $= 6.24 \times 10^{5}$ MeV

1 joule $= 10^{7}$ ergs

1 gray (Gy) $= 1$ J/kg $= 100$ rads

1 rad $= 100$ ergs/gm $= 0.01$ J/kg $= 0.01$ Gy

1 amu $= 931.14$ MeV

1 proton mass $= 938.21$ MeV $= 1.6724 \times 10^{-24}$ gm

1 neutron mass $= 939.50$ MeV $= 1.6747 \times 10^{-24}$ gm

1 electron mass $= 0.511$ MeV $= 9.108 \times 10^{-28}$ gm

Avogadro's number $= 6.023 \times 10^{23}$ atoms per mole

Velocity of light $= 3 \times 10^{10}$ cm/sec

Planck's constant $= 6.625 \times 10^{-27}$ erg-sec

# Appendix III

PHYSICAL DATA FOR SOME USEFUL RADIONUCLIDES

| Radionuclide | Mode of Decay | Half-Life | Principle Photon Energy keV |
|---|---|---|---|
| Carbon-11 | $\beta^+$ | 20.3 m | 511 |
| Nitrogen-13 | $\beta^+$ | 10 m | 511 |
| Oxygen-15 | $\beta^+$ | 2 m | 511 |
| Fluorine-18 | $\beta^+$ | 109 m | 511 |
| Potassium-43 | $\beta^-$ | 22.4 h | 619, 374 |
| Scandium-43 | $\beta^+$ | 3.9 h | 511 |
| Titanium-45 | $\beta^+$ | 3.1 h | 511 |
| Scandium-47 | $\beta^-$ | 3.4 d | 160 |
| Vanadium-47 | $\beta^+$ | 33 m | 511 |
| Cromium-51 | EC | 27.8 d | 320 |
| Cobalt-57 | EC | 270 d | 122 |
| Copper-67 | $\beta^-$ | 59 h | 184 |
| Gallium-67 | EC | 78 h | 184, 296 |
| Gallium-68 | $\beta^+$, EC | 68 m | 511 |
| Zinc-69m | IT, $\beta^-$ | 13.8 h | 439 |
| Selenium-75 | EC | 120 d | 136, 265 |
| Selenium-81m | IT, $\beta^-$ | 57 m | 103 |
| Rubidium-81 | EC, $\beta^+$ | 4.7 h | 190 |
| Strontium-87m | IT | 2.8 h | 388 |
| Ruthenium-97 | EC | 2.9 d | 215 |

| Radionuclide | Mode of Decay | Half-Life | Principle Photon Energy keV |
|---|---|---|---|
| Molybdenum-99 | $\beta^-$ | 67 h | 140, 740 |
| Technetium-99m | IT | 6 h | 140 |
| Indium-111 | EC | 2.8 d | 173, 247 |
| Indium-113m | IT | 100 m | 393 |
| Tin-117m | IT | 14 d | 158 |
| Antimony-117 | EC, $\beta^+$ | 2.8 h | 158 |
| Iodine-123 | EC | 13.3 h | 159 |
| Iodine-125 | EC | 60 d | 27 |
| Iodine-131 | $\beta^-$ | 8 d | 364 |
| Cesium-129 | EC | 32 h | 375, 416 |
| Xenon-127 | EC | 36.4 d | 203 |
| Xenon-133 | $\beta^-$ | 5.27 d | 29, 81 |
| Barium-135m | IT | 28.7 h | 268 |
| Cerium-141 | $\beta^-$ | 33 d | 145 |
| Dysprosium-157 | EC | 8.1 h | 326 |
| Erbium-165 | EC | 10.3 h | 50 |
| Thulium-167 | EC | 9.6 d | 208 |
| Yetterbium-169 | EC | 32 d | 198 |
| Tantulum-177 | EC | 56.6 h | 55 |
| Tantulum-180m | EC, $\beta^-$ | 8.7 h | 55 |
| Platinum-195m | IT | 4.1 d | 67 |
| Gold-196 | EC, $\beta^-$ | 6.18 d | 356 |
| Mercury-197 | EC | 65 h | 70 |
| Thallium-201 | EC | 73 h | 70 |
| Lead-203 | EC | 52.1 h | 280 |

# Appendix IV

ANSWERS TO QUESTIONS AND PROBLEMS

Chapter 1
 1. C 2. B 3. B 4. A 5. D 6. A 7. B 8. C 9. B 10. C

Chapter 2
 1. D 2. C 3. B 4. B 5. A 6. D 7. B 8. C 9. D 10. D

Chapter 3
 1. C 2. B 3. D 4. C 5. D 6. C 7. A 8. B 9. C 10. B
 11. C 12. C

Chapter 4
 1. C 2. C 3. C 4. A 5. B 6. C 7. A 8. B 9. D 10. A
 11. C 12. D 13.C 14.B

Chapter 5
 1. C 2. D 3. B 4. C 5. C 6. B 7. D

Chapter 6
 1. C 2. A 3. C 4. B 5. D

Chapter 7
 1. D 2. B 3. B 4. B 5. C 6. B 7. C

Chapter 8
 1. D 2. B 3. B 4. D 5. A 6. B 7. A 8. C 9. D

Chapter 9
 1. D 2. B 3. B 4. B 5. B 6. D 7. D 8. D

Chapter 10
 1. B 2. A 3. D 4. C 5. A 6. C 7. C 8. A 9. D 10. A

Chapter 11

1. B    2. B    3. C    4. C    5. A    6. D    7. D    8. C    9. B    10. B
11. C

Chapter 12

1. A    2. C    3. D    4. D    5. D    6. C    7. B    8. C    9. B    10. C

# Index